MW01592196

INTERMITTENT FASTING 101

For Women who Desire to Purify their Body, Lose Weight and Slow Aging using 16/8 Method, Self-Cleaning Process of Autophagy and Keto Diet (3 Books in 1 with over 50 recipes)

Jennifer Cook

© **Jennifer Cook - Copyright 2020 - All rights reserved.**

The content contained within this book may not be reproduced, duplicated or transmitted without direct written permission from the author or the publisher.
Under no circumstances will any blame or legal responsibility be held against the publisher, or author, for any damages, reparation, or monetary loss due to the information contained within this book. Either directly or indirectly.

Legal Notice:
This book is copyright protected. This book is only for personal use. You cannot amend, distribute, sell, use, quote or paraphrase any part, or the content within this book, without the consent of the author or publisher.

Disclaimer Notice:
Please note the information contained within this document is for educational and entertainment purposes only. All effort has been executed to present accurate, up to date, and reliable, complete information. No warranties of any kind are declared or implied. Readers acknowledge that the author is not engaging in the rendering of legal, financial, medical or professional advice. The content within this book has been derived from various sources. Please consult a licensed professional before attempting any techniques outlined in this book.

By reading this document, the reader agrees that under no circumstances is the author responsible for any losses, direct or indirect, which are incurred as a result of the use of information contained within this document, including, but not limited to, — errors, omissions, or inaccuracies.

This book Includes:

Autophagy

For Women and Men who Desire to Purify their Body, Lose Weight, and Slow Aging with a Natural Self-Cleaning Metabolic Process using Extended Water, Intermittent Fasting and a Ketogenic Diet

Intermittent Fasting for Women 101

The Ultimate Step-by-Step Guide for Weight Loss, Even If You Are Over 50, with the Keto Diet, 16/8 Method and Self-Cleansing Through the Metabolic Process of Autophagy

Intermittent Fasting Diet Guide

A Complete Step-By-Step Guide for Heal Your Body, Weight Loss, Fat Burn and Live in a Healthy and Happy Way with the Autophagy Process
(Meal Plan with 60 Recipes)

By
Jennifer Cook

Table of Contents

Autophagy _____ **13**

Introduction _____ 14

Chapter 1: Autophagy Process - Code of Longevity
_____ 16

The Biology behind Autophagy's Anti-Aging Effects__ 19

Correcting Myths about Autophagy and Anti-Aging __ 21

How Different Means of Turning On Autophagy Affect
Anti-Aging _____ 23

The Newest Findings in Biology Concerning Autophagy
and the Fight against Aging_____ 26

Chapter 2: What We Know about Autophagy So Far
_____ 28

Micro, Macro, and Chaperone-Mediated Autophagy__ 30

The Biology of Autophagy_____ 38

Chapter 3: Why Intermittent Fasting _____ 43

Starting your First Intermittent Fast _____ 51

Protein Cycling during Intermittent Fasting _____ 53

Chapter 4: Keto Diet _____ 57

The Mechanisms of Keto _____ 61

Keto: The Practical Walkthrough _____ 65

Chapter 5: Extended Water Fasting _____ 71

Water Fasting: a Practical Walkthrough _____ 76

Inside the Mind of a Person doing a Water Fast _____ 81

Chapter 6: Metabolic Autophagy Foods _____ 84

Eating Right for Autophagy _____ 85

Chapter 7: Metabolic Autophagy in Practice _____ 98

What to Avoid in Your First Fast _____ 102

Chapter 8: Autophagy and Training to Build Muscle _____ 110

The Health of the Individual who Exercises to Increase Autophagy _____ 113

A Note before the Conclusion _____ 119

Conclusion _____ 121

Appendix: Scientific studies on autophagy, intermittent fasting and related subjects _____ 124

Intermittent Fasting for Women 101 128

Introduction _____ 129

Chapter 1 _____ 132

The American Woman who Wants to Lose Weight _____ 132

A Broad Look at How an American Woman Can Lose Weight with Intermittent Fasting _____ 135

Intermittent Fasting as an Alternative to Less Healthy Methods that May Not Even Work _____ 142

Chapter 2 _____ 144

What is Intermittent Fasting? _____ 144

Intermittent Fasting: Looking at its Effects on Health More Closely _____ 147

Intermittent Fasting and Autophagy _____158

The Ideal Diet for a Woman Doing Intermittent Fasting
_____161

Your Options for Different Methods of Intermittent
Fasting _____168

Chapter 3: _____*171*

Benefits of Intermittent Fasting _____*171*

Autophagy: Nature's Detoxifier _____171

Autophagy and Your Skin _____175

Autophagy and Your Energy _____181

Autophagy: It's What's Good for You_____183

Chapter 4 _ _____*188*

*Intermittent Fasting and Autophagy*_____*188*

Where It All Started _____190

Micro-autophagy_____192

Macro-autophagy _____192

Chaperone-Mediated Autophagy _____193

Microscopic is Everything _____197

The Newest Science _____202

*Chapter 5*_____*205*

Food to Eat During Intermittent Fasting _____*205*

*Chapter 6*_____*217*

Intermittent Fasting and Women _____*217*

Intermittent Fasting and Women: Made for Each Other
_____220

Chapter 7: _____ 223

Intermittent Fasting for Women over 50 _____ 223

Chapter 8 Intermittent Fasting Techniques: 16/8, Keto Diet, and More _____ 231

The 12-Hour Fast _____ 233

The 8-Hour Fast _____ 234

The 5:2 Fast _____ 235

Concurrent Day Fasting _____ 236

Conclusion _____ 238

Appendix: Studies on Intermittent Fasting and Autophagy _____ 241

INTERMITTENT FASTING DIET GUIDE   **244**

Introduction _____ 247

Chapter 1 Intermittent Fasting _____ 249

What Is Fasting? _____ 249

What Is Intermittent Fasting? _____ 250

Intermittent Fasting And Weight Loss _____ 251

How Intermittent Fasting Helps To Lose Weight? __ 252

Chapter 2 Intermittent Fasting Benefits _____ 254

How Intermittent Fasting Helps? _____ 254

Health Benefits _____ 257

Intermittent Fasting & Obesity _____ 259

Chapter 3 Who Can Do Fasting? _____ 262

Guide For Kids _____ 262

Intermittent Fasting And Women _____264

Fasting And Diabetics_____267

Bottom Line _____268

Chapter 4 Intermittent Fasting With Keto Diet___270

Keto Diet & Its Health Benefits_____270

Do's & Don'ts In Keto Diet _____272

Keto Diet With Intermittent Fasting & Weight Loss _275

Chapter 5 Metabolic Autophagy _____277

How Does Autophagy Work?_____277

Diet Should Follow Autophagy: _____283

Metabolic Disorders & Autophagy _____ _____284

Chapter 6 Intermittent Fasting 101 Methods ____288

Advantages Of Intermittent Fasting: _____289

16:8 Fasting Method_____290

What Is 20:4? _____292

Long Fasts_____293

Fast Diet – 5:2 _____294

24 & 36 Hours Fasting _____296

Fasting In Alternative Days _____298

Impulsive Fasting_____299

Warrior Fasting _____300

Protein Sparing Modified Fasting (PSMF) _____303

Bottom Line _____305

Chapter 7 How To Start With Intermittent Fasting?
_____306

How To Start Intermittent Fasting?_____ 307

Benefits Of Following The Fasting _____ 308

Things To Consider Before Starting_____ 309

Chapter 8 Intermittent Fasting And Workout ___ 311

Fasting And Gain Muscle _____ 312

Effects On Men & Women Physique_____ 314

Best Exercise During Intermittent Fasting _____ 316

Chapter 9 Tips For Successful Transformation__ 319

Motivational Success Stories _____ 320

Tips For Transformation_____ 323

Chapter 10 Women And Intermittent Fasting ___ 328

During Mensuration _____ 330

For Pregnancy & Breastfeeding_____ 331

During Menopause _____ 332

The Best Methods Of Intermittent Fasting For Women ___ 334

Chapter 11: Recipes_____ 337

Raspberry Power Pancake _____ 337

Chocolate Chip Whey Waffles _____ 339

Cinnamon Sugar Donuts _____ 340

Poached Eggs & Avocado _____ 341

Chocolate Chia Plain Pudding _____ 343

Gluten-Free Pumpkin Pancake _____ 344

Roasted Sweet Potato & Poblano Tacos _____ 345

Sugar-Free Oatmeal Cookies_____ 346

Egg Muffin With Broccoli_____ 348

Banana Blueberry Muffins _____349

Grilled Cheeseburger _____351

Asian Chicken Salad _____352

Keto Chicken Lettuce Wraps _____353

Egg And Vegetable Bagel Sandwich _____355

Chicken Caprese Sandwich_____356

Slow-Cooker Split Pea Soup _____357

Cobb Egg Salad _____359

Chicken Cheese Sandwich _____360

Charred Shrimp And Avocado_____362

Grilled Steak Tortilla _____363

One-Pot Beef With Broccoli _____365

Sheet Pan Sausages & Veggies _____366

Loaded Sheet Pan Nachos _____367

Lemon & Garlic Salmon With Asparagus _____369

Slow Cooker BBQ Chicken _____370

Crispy Cauliflower Tacos _____371

Chicken Scampi Pasta _____372

Chicken Steak With Stuffed Potatoes_____375

Buffalo Chicken Enchiladas_____376

Hot Sausages Cast-Iron Skillet Pan Pizza _____378

Potato Lollipop_____380

Potato Cheese Balls_____381

Crispy Pepperoni Chips _____382

Candied Almonds _____384

Wheat Crackers _____ 385

Cranberry Nut Granola Bar _____ 387

Bacon Avocado Fries _____ 388

Jalapeno Popper Crisps _____ 389

Peanut Butter Protein Balls _____ 390

Veggies Cheese Rolls _____ 391

Strawberry Smoothie _____ 393

Caramel Popcorn _____ 394

Chocolate Chip Cookies _____ 395

Granola Bars _____ 396

Nutella Sandwich _____ 397

Oreo Truffles _____ 399

Chocolate Covered Cake Balls _____ 400

Pumpkin Cake Roll _____ 401

Peanut Butter No-Bake Cookies _____ 402

Apple Pie _____ 403

Choco & Fruit Mousse _____ 406

Chocolate Smoothie _____ 407

Grilled Cheese Bites _____ 408

Chopped Chickpea Salad _____ 409

Frozen Berry Yogurt _____ 411

Choco Bombs _____ 412

Chocolate Chip Muffins _____ 413

Cinnamon cupcake _____ 414

Mixed Fruit Trifle _____ 416

Carrot Cake Bliss Balls_____417

Chapter 12 21day Meal Plan _____*419*

Chapter 13 Faqs _____*425*

Conclusion _____*433*

Autophagy

For Women and Men who Desire to Purify their Body, Lose Weight, and Slow Aging with a Natural Self-Cleaning Metabolic Process using Extended Water, Intermittent Fasting and a Ketogenic Diet.

Jennifer Cook

Introduction

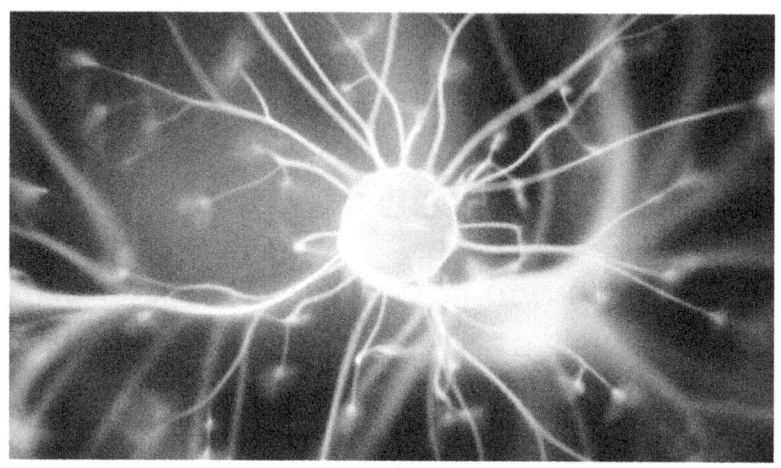

Congratulations on purchasing *Autophagy,* and thank you for doing so.

With the serious problem of obesity all over the world, not just in the United States, it is understandable that people are looking for a scientifically proven way to lose weight. Turning on autophagy in your body fits the bill perfectly. Read our comprehensive guidebook to the world of autophagy and how you can use its healing potential to lose weight, combat aging, and feel young.

Autophagy is at the center of the changes you can make in your daily life to see these effects. Put simply, autophagy is your cells' natural detoxifier. It is a natural biological process that has existed since the first single-celled organisms came to be on Earth.

Humans in the first world have lost touch with the process of autophagy because of the onset of industrialized agriculture and the resulting abundance of food. Not so long ago, we as a species went through long spans of time without eating. We didn't do this for the health benefits — we did it because we didn't have any food.

In the past, when people went through days without eating, our bodies started the process of autophagy in the cells. Since we did not have food in our cells for them to consume, our cells found alternate sources of energy to break down, such as damaged organelles, protein clumps, and various toxins. Autophagy gave us the twofold benefit of decluttering our cells and filling us with energy.

Of course, autophagy never totally went away. It is just that we don't go through it as much since we are constantly eating. Our book will teach you how to energize autophagy in your body so you can feel young, look young, and lose weight.

There are plenty of books on this subject on the market, thanks again for choosing this one! Every effort was made to ensure it is full of as much useful information as possible; please enjoy!

Chapter 1
Autophagy Process - Code of Longevity

As the years go by and you go through the natural process of aging, a lot of changes happen in your body. Your skin loses its stretchiness, you gain weight more easily, and you start to feel tired more often. Autophagy is your best friend in fighting against these processes so you can look and feel young for longer. Take the effect of autophagy on your skin. Turning autophagy on in your skin cells will allow them to produce more collagen, a protein produced by your fibroblasts, a type of cell in your skin.

Collagen is the protein that makes your skin stretchier and more youthful. It will put your cells in a routine of cleaning themselves out more so they can work more efficiently, making you feel more active and engaged with the world. This is just one of the benefits of higher autophagy in your body. The benefits of autophagy are innumerable, and it is never too late to learn more about them.

Until now, you've gone about dieting the wrong way. There are many diets that help you lose weight for a short time, but they're bad for your body, and they don't help you keep the weight off in the long term. This is what makes an autophagy-centered health routine so different from following fat diets. Autophagy is a method of keeping weight off your body while also considering your overall health — because you don't just want to lose weight. You want what is best for your general health.

There's also good news in the fact that for women especially, a lower BMI (proportion of fat to body mass) is a good indicator of your overall health. That might not be surprising to you; if you have ever been to the doctor after losing weight, it is unlikely they expressed concern over your weight. In today's society, in particular, many people struggle to keep their weight down. Doing so isn't just a matter of looking better — it is a legitimate indicator of your health.

Overweight and obese people have higher risks of heart disease, stroke, and more as they age. On the other hand, thinner people are not looking at these same risks. Losing weight can only be good for your body, and autophagy is the healthiest and most effective way to do it. Autophagy will help you stay thin, feel good, and be healthy for years and years.

But so far, we have only talked about the health benefits that are immediately obvious. There is also a reduction of health risks that are not cosmetic, like youthful skin and weight loss. It has been proven that an increase in autophagy reduces your risk of Alzheimer's and Parkinson's disease. More autophagy also reduces inflammation, which will increase your overall health. There has even been research about the benefits of autophagy for cancer patients undergoing chemotherapy.

Studies have shown that cancer patients going through chemotherapy saw a reduction in the clumps of white blood cells that accumulate because of chemotherapy. Dead cells can be hazardous to your body if they are not cleaned out during autophagy. Since these patients fasted in order to turn on autophagy, their bodies were able to clean out the white blood cells and recover from chemotherapy sooner.

You can only imagine the kind of advantage you get if you are turning autophagy on as much as possible, and you aren't even looking at a major health risk yet. You may not have as big an accumulation of dead cells as someone going through chemotherapy, but if you have not fasted before and you don't exercise regularly, it is very likely that you have a lot of toxins in your body. This is because if you don't go through autophagy very often, materials like dead cells, dead organelles, and unused proteins start to pile up and make your cells less efficient.

Putting your body through autophagy doesn't just combat aging in ways that are immediately visible. It also greatly reduces your risk of long-term age-related disease. Whether you're looking to improve the quality of your life or the length of your life, making autophagy happen in your body will do it.

You can also feel relief in the fact that the book you are reading contains all you need to know about autophagy and how to best manipulate it for your health. After experiencing the life-changing effects of increased autophagy and consulting countless scientific journals on the subject, I know what information about autophagy you don't want to miss.

The Biology behind Autophagy's Anti-Aging Effects

Behind all the positive health consequences that come from autophagy is the biology that makes it work. As the pioneering biologist behind the biggest discoveries on the topic, Yoshinori Ohsumi underlined the importance of a process called cell recycling. Most books about autophagy tell us about the way our cells discard toxins, but they do not go into what our cells do with these broken down components.

It is not just toxin disposal that makes autophagy so good for us, but also cell recycling, so it's vital for you to know how it works. Scientists are still trying to understand some of the more intricate parts of autophagy, but they can tell us the basic mechanisms at play.

First, the cells must be put into a state of stress. This is where fasting and other methods of autophagy stimulation come in. These methods put your cells into a state of stress and activate autophagy. When they are under stress, autophagy begins with the structure called the autophagosome. The autophagosome travels inside the cell looking for things it can break down for nutrients, including all the things we have talked about so far: unused proteins, unused organelles, and other toxins that come from outside the cell.

The next step is where a cellular structure called the lysosome comes in. While you can think of the autophagosome as the transporter to the cell stomach, you can see the lysosome as the cell stomach itself. Back when the French scientist Christian De Duve discovered the lysosome in the 60s, we thought the lysosome was the cell's garbage receptacle; we did not know at the time that it was more like a recycling bin. The autophagosome takes all the materials it finds and binds with the lysosome, so these materials can be broken down for reuse.

There are multiple autophagosomes in your body, by the way, and the longer you are in a state of stress from starvation, the more you will have. More autophagosomes means more autophagy in your body. Research has concluded that you get the highest number of autophagosomes after 36 hours of fasting and that you do not see more autophagosomes after this point.

Of course, we are doing a little bit of simplification, but the next step is essentially the last step of autophagy. Even the microbiologists simplify things when they discuss autophagy because they don't know everything about this process either — the finer points of autophagy are still being worked out. The newest discoveries about autophagy are concerned with this third and final stage. In it, your cells take the broken down parts they obtained through autophagy and use them to build new organelles and protein structures.

Technically, this is not the final stage of autophagy, because by this time, autophagy has finished and your cells are no longer in a state of stress. This stage is the most exciting for people who care about advancements in science that have implications in health and anti-aging because with this stage we aren't just talking about detoxifying your body.

We are talking about using the fine materials gained from the detox for rebuilding cellular structures. When your cells use these broken down components to build new structures, your body has new, young structures at the lowest level, and this is a very exciting opportunity for your health.

When your cells have newly-built parts, they run more smoothly, live longer, and keep your body running efficiently. With autophagy, you get two great benefits in one: the removal of microscopic waste that would eventually turn toxic, and the repurposing of this microscopic junk into new, young cell parts that do a lot of good in changing your body into a healthy one.

To remember the stages of autophagy, think of the first stage as the autophagosome stage, the second as the lysosome stage, and the third as cell recycling. In few words, the process of autophagy involves the autophagosome collecting waste, the lysosome breaking down waste, and the cell using the parts left over to build new structures.

Correcting Myths about Autophagy and Anti-Aging

There are many misconceptions about how autophagy does its anti-aging work. Perhaps the most common is that its only health benefits come from taking care of toxins. Clearing toxins from your system is certainly a good thing, but autophagy goes far beyond ridding your body of harmful chemicals. Most of these toxins are not from outside your body, but they are materials like proteins and organelles that your cells used once and then no longer had a use for. These discarded materials start to take up space over time, creating clutter that slows down your cells. This is when they become toxins.

Some of these toxins cause even worse problems than congestion. The worst case is protein clusters that form in the brain. Neurodegenerative diseases like Alzheimer's become more of a concern as we age, and autophagy might be your best ally in fighting against your risk of these diseases. From a broader perspective, Alzheimer's manifests as "knots" and "tangles" in the brain that impair memory.

When doctors look at the knots and tangles with a microscope, they see that these irregularities are actually clusters of proteins that have built up over time. They are proteins that brain cells used at one point but later had no purpose. The protein clusters were not managed with autophagy, so they simply accumulated and started leading to serious memory problems.

Alzheimer's disease is the most extreme consequence that you can have from not going through enough autophagy. It is not the only consequence, however. Discarded materials like protein clusters start to build up throughout your body if you rarely go through autophagy.

In this regard, low autophagy leads to a low count of collagen, the protein that makes your skin youthful. Your skin cells can't produce collagen when they are crowded by cellular garbage. Similarly, you lose more muscle mass if you rarely go through autophagy because you are not turning on autophagy to repair the muscle tissue damage that results from physical activity.

From these examples alone, you can see that autophagy is more than a toxin-cleaning agent. Autophagy doesn't only destroy the bad (toxins); it builds the good (new organelles, proteins, and cells). Both sides of autophagy make it such a powerful anti-aging tool, one that was surprisingly given to us by nature.

So far, we have established that autophagy isn't just good for destroying pathogen invaders — it also destroys materials that become toxic when they linger in the cell for too long. In short, this biological process cleans out toxins from the outside and inside.

In the third stage, your cells use these broken down parts as ingredients to build new cells and cell structures. What's more: your cells have more room to build new cells and new cell parts because they freed up so much space during autophagy.

All these things come together when you find a way to turn on autophagy on a regular basis. Equipped with all this information, you know much more about autophagy than even your average fasting practitioner.

How Different Means of Turning On Autophagy Affect Anti-Aging

We will go deep into every method and how they start up the process of autophagy in different ways. To start out, let's just talk about what these methods are and how each of them combats aging in their own way.

The most well-known method is fasting. There are several different types of fasting, including intermittent fasting, water fasting, concurrent day fasting, and more. What makes fasting, so reliable is that you don't have to do something new, you just have to stop doing something that you are already doing. To turn on autophagy with exercise, you have to get into a new routine of working out regularly, and with the keto diet, you have to start a new way of eating.

In order to fast, you just have to refrain from eating when you would normally eat. We have already gone over the health benefits that come from autophagy, but with fasting, you also get health benefits from simply consuming fewer calories.

Back in the 90s, the idea of caloric restriction became very popular, and people saw improvements in their health from doing nothing more than eating less. There is even a great deal of evidence that mammals who restrict their calories live longer than mammals who do not.

This has not yet been proven to be true for humans, but still, restricting your caloric intake can only be a good thing. You get this additional benefit from turning on autophagy through fasting while also getting the benefit of autophagy itself along with it.

We have heard a lot of ideas about losing weight from nutritionists in the last few decades, but let's not kid ourselves: the main reason for weight gain across the planet comes down to people consuming a lot of calories without physically exerting themselves to burn them off. Fasting for any length of time will lead to consuming fewer calories, so you are on the right track for losing weight when you fast.

The next popular method of turning on autophagy is the keto diet. This method will turn on autophagy because it involves depriving your body of nutrients that it would normally consume for energy.

However, following the keto diet alone will not turn on autophagy because it is only activated when your cells are in a state of stress, and as long as you are sedentary or filling your body with any kind of food, your cells are not in this state.

That said, since the keto diet is so low in carbs, this style of eating will aid in turning on autophagy. I definitely recommend following the keto diet because the mistake many autophagy practitioners make is consuming a lot of carbs while they are not fasting.

Eating a lot of carbs will prevent your body from fasting for a long time because it takes a long time for your digestive system to process them. Not only that, but as you may be aware, it becomes harder to keep weight off the older you get, and you are significantly slowing down the process of burning fat when your digestive tract has a backlog of carbs. Fighting against this problem is the role of the keto diet in anti-aging and autophagy.

Next, there is the method of exercise. Studies have shown that resistance training, also known as strength training, is the most effective way of turning on autophagy, saying it is even more effective than fasting. The reason for this is that when you use your muscles, you are getting tiny tears in your muscle tissue that are repaired through autophagy.

The unfortunate thing is that exercising might be the last thing that people want to do, even though it is so good for their health. Like the other methods, exercise has its own health benefits that are separate from autophagy. Plenty of studies show that people who work out regularly have lower risks of all age-related illnesses, even those not related to the heart. If we are honest, exercising is probably the best way to fight aging.

If you want to get the most out of autophagy, you should employ all of these methods together. When combined, the keto diet, exercise, and fasting will give you the greatest benefits, both in terms of weight loss and in general health.

If you don't yet feel motivated to be as healthy as possible, try to think of the autophagy in your cells as an analogy for your personal health. If they did not recycle their cellular garbage, your cells would simply die after their organelles stopped working, or they were overcrowded with protein clusters and foreign invaders.

If you do not recycle your body's toxins by turning on autophagy regularly, your body will be over-encumbered with cellular garbage, and you will be less healthy as a result. If this analogy were expanded, you might even live a shorter life if you do not regularly clean out your cellular garbage via autophagy. Your cells try to live longer by using autophagy to combat their cellular aging — you should try to use autophagy to work against aging too.

The Newest Findings in Biology Concerning Autophagy and the Fight against Aging

Some of the recent findings about autophagy have turned out to be incredibly relevant to matters of personal health. It has only been in the past decade that we found out that Alzheimer's and Parkinson's disease are a result of a mutation in a gene that controls autophagy.

Let's step back for a second and define what we mean by mutation. As we age, the DNA in our cells becomes damaged from wear and tear. One of the genes in our DNA is the one that controls autophagy. When that gene takes damage, our autophagy is less effective because it is not getting proper instructions from the DNA.

As a result, when your brain cells create protein chains to do certain jobs, these protein chains become clusters that are toxic to your cells, all because these cells did not have undamaged genes from which to take their instructions.

Now you might worry that this gene damage as a result of age means that there is nothing you can do about it, but this could not be further from the truth. Your takeaway from this scientific discovery should be that you need to manually turn on autophagy as you get older because your cells' genes will not be as effective at doing it automatically. You can turn on autophagy through fasting, the keto diet, or exercise and get the same much-needed autophagy as you would if your genes instructed your cells to do it to themselves.

Chapter 2
What We Know about Autophagy So Far

Biologists used to think an organelle in cells called the lysosome was no more than a trash dispenser. It wasn't until the earth-shattering discoveries of scientist Yoshinori Ohsumi that we found out that the lysosome was the base of one of the body's most elaborate functions at the microscopic level. Put simply, autophagy is when your body's cells have no food from the outside, so they trap toxins, unused organelles, and discarded proteins in the lysosome.

The lysosome breaks down these materials into parts that the cell and build into something new. We have already covered these basic facts about autophagy, but it's good to review them to make sure we are on the same page.

When Ohsumi looked into autophagy with a tiny group of scientists, there were not many who were interested in the subject. Ever since winning the Nobel Prize, however, more biologists have woken up to how fascinating the subject is.

The group of researchers started out looking at autophagy in yeast cells in the 60s, and even today, they are still looking at yeast cells because there are still aspects of autophagy they do not understand. In science, it is best to use the same case to learn more about something, and for autophagy, they use the yeast cell as their case.

In an interview, Ohsumi has said he felt that they still only understand about 30% of the process of autophagy.

Even if they only come to understand autophagy 50% of the way, there is a good chance that these findings will be miraculous for people living with cancer or age-related diseases. The best part is that even armed with 30% of our modern understanding of autophagy, you can make changes to your daily routine that will help you live longer and lose weight. Still, it is exciting that scientists could find something revelatory by looking at yeast cells' autophagy that could change medicine completely.

We have discussed the fact that autophagy has been shown to be related to neurodegenerative diseases like Alzheimer's and Parkinson's, but those are not the only diseases that it may play a key role in. There has been cutting edge research showing that when you put cancer cells (of a disease like neuroblastoma) in a petri dish with drugs that stimulate autophagy, those cancer cells are shown to have inhibited growth. In this case, the cancer cells were put together in a dish with a drug called apocynin, and the cancer cells had less growth because of the drug that stimulated autophagy.

This should be taken with a grain of salt because there has actually been research showing that autophagy can speed the growth of cancer cells as well — it just depends on the specific situation. But this is getting too far into the scientific details. The main takeaway for you is that autophagy plays an important, irreplaceable role throughout the body, and while your body is basically healthy, you cannot do wrong by stimulating it as much as you can.

In the following section, we will talk about the three kinds of autophagy that we know about so far. Before we do so, though, we want to clarify what we mean by "stress" in this book. There is a big difference between the kind of stress you put on your cell to turn on autophagy and the psychological stress that you might feel while you're approaching a deadline at work.

You do not have to feel psychological stress to turn on autophagy; you just need to put your cells under acute stress by depriving of nutrients or through exercise. If you do that, they will eat their cellular garbage in order to survive.

Micro, Macro, and Chaperone-Mediated Autophagy

Scientists know about three kinds of autophagy: microautophagy, macroautophagy, and chaperone-mediated autophagy. Microautophagy occurs in every cell of your body, so it is the most common. Meanwhile, macroautophagy happens only in specialized cells such as white blood cells.

Chaperone-mediated autophagy is the kind that scientists are studying the most because it has wide health implications that could potentially cure age-related disease or cancer. When scientists found out that Alzheimer's and Parkinson's were a result of failed autophagy because of damaged genes, these genes were actually instructions for chaperone-mediated autophagy.

This specific finding brought autophagy to the attention of scientists at large. There are now many researchers looking into the intricacies of chaperone-mediated autophagy.

Microautophagy happens in every cell with a lysosome — that is, every cell in your body. I told you before that the autophagosome brings in cellular garbage to the lysosome, but that was just to keep things simple. The autophagosome is only used for macroautophagy. In most cells, only microautophagy is performed, and the lysosome simply pulls in the cellular garbage on its own, without the help of an autophagosome.

Microautophagy has several purposes. Every cell goes through this process to maintain equilibrium in the membrane, to survive when low on nutrients, and to maintain the size of organelles such as the mitochondria.

Scientists have looked inside the lysosome during microautophagy to see how exactly the materials are broken down, and they found that enzymes are sent into the lysosome to attack the toxins.

Once this process is complete, the broken down materials are used for fatty acids, amino acids, and so on. This is all part of the essential process all cells go through in order to survive, called the cell cycle. Becoming familiar with the cell cycle should help you visualize yourself as a cell that must constantly renew itself through autophagy, just as your cells do.

Now let's talk about macroautophagy, the kind of autophagy that is not seen in most cells, only in one with special jobs like white blood cells. This is the kind of autophagy that uses autophagosomes, which leave the cell to find materials like protein clumps, damaged organelles, and foreign toxins.

The jelly-like substance around the cell and inside cells is called cytoplasm, and the autophagosome has to take in materials from the cytoplasm and carry them over to the lysosome.

The lysosome is where the process of macroautophagy starts looking exactly like the process of microautophagy. When the autophagosome moves the materials into the lysosome, that part of the process is named by scientists' sequestration.

The other difference between macroautophagy and microautophagy is that in macroautophagy, the lysosome does not breakdown the materials. In macroautophagy, this is the autophagosome's job. The autophagosome binds with the lysosome to break down the materials.

The other name for macroautophagy is phagocytosis. The word phagocytosis is generally the term used for when cells run into a large particle from outside, and then surround it with the autophagosome to keep it under control. After that, the same procedure occurs, and the large particle is moved to the lysosome, where the materials are broken down.

The autophagosome is the special organelle that makes macroautophagy a little different from the other kinds of autophagy. Technically speaking, the autophagosome is not considered an organelle, but a vesicle. It is not truly an organelle because it is not a structure that supports the basic functions of a cell, but rather it is a tool that the cell builds to perform a task outside of the cell. As you know, the job of the autophagosome is to find materials to break down in the lysosome. It secures these materials with its double-membrane so they cannot escape.

The last major kind of autophagy is called chaperone-mediated autophagy. This is the newest type that anyone is aware of. In chaperone-mediated autophagy, the lysosome and the autophagosome do not work alone; they work with specialized protein chains. These protein chains have a job: to move particular particles into the cell stomach (lysosome). In other words, chaperone-mediated autophagy is not for getting rid of just any cellular garbage as in microautophagy. Chaperone-mediated autophagy is looking for specific particles using these specialized protein chains and bringing them into the lysosome for breakdown.

This is the kind of autophagy that scientists are trying to learn about the most since it is the most linked to certain diseases. It has been postulated that this kind of autophagy may be essential for the prevention of disease since it can use protein chains to find specific kinds of particles that can be broken down for specific raw materials, in order to build up specific structures. These specific cellular structures may be able to stave off disease.

So far in the lab, chaperone-mediated autophagy has been shown to play an essential role in repairing genes, in the breakdown of particles, and keeping the level of glucose at equilibrium. Chaperone-mediated autophagy is most similar to the process of microautophagy. The difference is that it does not break down just any content that it finds inside or outside the cell.

With microautophagy, the cell breaks down anything that is hindering its work as a cell. With chaperone-mediated autophagy, the cell is looking for specific content in the cytoplasm. The cell's genes contain instructions on what materials to break down in the process of chaperone-mediated autophagy.

With all this talk about how important chaperone-mediated autophagy is, you might be tempted to think microautophagy and macroautophagy are less important. But if you want to be healthy, lose weight, and feel better, it's important to turn on autophagy of all kinds because they all maintain the health of your body.

To be sure, chaperone-mediated autophagy is the most exciting kinds of autophagy to study for scientists. It is an established fact by this point that chaperone-mediated is highly linked to diseases that come with old age, especially as a result of neurodegeneration. There has also been a clear link made between cancer and a failure of chaperone-mediated autophagy.

As we have discussed before, this failure is the result of the degradation of genes that comes from aging. These are the genes that are meant to tell your cells to go through chaperone-mediated autophagy. When your cells do not have instructions from this gene to tell them to start chaperone-mediated autophagy, they do not, so protein chains build up and create toxins, particularly in your brain. This is why manually turning on autophagy through fasting, diet, and exercise is so important.

The proteins used in chaperone-mediated autophagy are called chaperone proteins, which is what chaperone-mediated autophagy gets its name from. Your cells use these chaperone proteins to bring waste materials into the lysosome that the genes tell your cells are important to break down.

We know the least about chaperone-mediated autophagy because it is the latest one that we have discovered, but it is also the most important to research for scientists because of its serious health implications.

Autophagy is constantly happening in your body, so when we talk about activating or turning on autophagy, we are not saying that it is not going on at all in the first place. When we say turn it on, we mean increase it. Your cells will go through autophagy no matter what, but the scale of autophagy is what is important.

The truth is that the cells in your body are going through autophagy right now, at this very moment, somewhere. But if you exercise, more follow the ketogenic diet, and fast, the amount of autophagy will go way up.

For example, someone who developed Alzheimer's is still going through autophagy, and they did before they started getting symptoms of the disease, but if they had stimulated autophagy before the onset of Alzheimer's, they may not have ended up getting it, because their cells would have been spurred to take care of the protein clumps that lead to the disease.

The research even shows that your cells reach a peak of chaperone-mediated autophagy after 10 hours of fasting. That means if you want to get some of the benefit of this special kind of autophagy, then you should aim to fast for at least ten hours, which is something that everyone is capable of.

That said, you still want to go further than that to unleash the full potential of this biological process, so you should ideally start with the ten-hour fast and work up to longer ones such as the water fast. We will get to the details of different kinds of fasts later on in the book.

It is quite exciting that chaperone-mediated autophagy only takes 10 hours of fasting to start up significantly, because it may be the most important kind of autophagy for you to turn on. Every type of autophagy will play an essential role in the cell cycle by getting rid of proteins that hinder the job of a cell. They will all involve reusing the raw materials from the dysfunctional proteins.

But chaperone-mediated autophagy is even more important because it purposefully and selectively gets rid of proteins that are harmful to your body, whereas the other types of autophagy will only remove these problematic proteins incidentally.

You can think of chaperone-mediated autophagy as the smart autophagy because microautophagy and macroautophagy do important work, but they only get rid of toxic protein build-up when they stumble upon it. In chaperone-mediated autophagy, your cells use the instructions in their genes to look out for and apprehend specific kinds of proteins that are bad for your cells.

Scientists have even named the special protein at the surface of the stomach that is used for chaperone-mediated autophagy, and it is called LAMP-2A. LAMP-2A is an abbreviation for lysosome-associated membrane protein. Part of the reason we know that this type of autophagy is so important is from research done on mice. One study found that when LAMP-2A was protected in mice, these mice lived healthier and longer lives than mice whose LAMP-2A was not protected.

If that doesn't convince you of the importance of LAMP-2A and chaperone-mediated autophagy, then I'm not sure what will. After all, it is just one protein at the end of the day, but it has such an outsized impact. The study suggests that we, as humans, should not underestimate the importance of autophagy in keeping us healthy. The importance of chaperone-mediated autophagy should not be underestimated either.

You may think there could not be possibly more good things about chaperone-mediated autophagy, but you would be wrong. There has been extensive research on it, and the findings are numerous. One of many similar studies showed that chaperone-mediated autophagy does not only have the function of breaking down specific proteins, but when done correctly, chaperone-mediated autophagy helps with glucose metabolism, and it can even help repair genes.

This is an especially important function since, as we have made clear, damaged genes can lead to a long list of diseases linked to aging. All of this is why scientists are interested in chaperone-mediated autophagy in particular.

In Parkinson's disease, in particular, researchers have found a connection with problems with chaperone-mediated autophagy. This problem happens because the proteins that are collected with chaperone-mediated autophagy bond with LAMP-2A too strongly, which causes clogging. It is clogging that leads to the protein build-up associated with Parkinson's disease.

You may be concerned that you already have a lot of protein buildup in your body, but no matter how far along this is, starting to turn on autophagy more will remedy the situation. Autophagy has numerous benefits: it will make your body's immune system better, it will prevent infection, cancer, and inflammation. These are just a few of the amazing benefits that autophagy has on your body as a whole.

The Biology of Autophagy

Your cells are the reason that your body is able to do anything. Even though they are so small that we can't even see them, you wouldn't be able to do any of the things that you do without your cells. Unfortunately, one of the most prominent features of aging is the degradation of your cells. Because of this, your cells' organelles are not as good when you are older.

The good thing is that you can turn on autophagy more so that aging does not affect your cells as much, and therefore they do not endure as much damage. When you do this, aging has less of an effect on you, and you will live longer than if you didn't activate it. If you are not turning on autophagy on a regular basis, your cells age and degrade much faster because you are not causing them to dispose of toxic elements as much, and as a result, they are full of toxins.

Your cells do not work nearly as well without autophagy: because of this, you are more susceptible to gain weight, having less youthful skin, having more inflamed pores, and having less energy. You are also more susceptible to diseases related to age.

As we have said before, the details are so complicated that even the smartest scientists are still trying to figure it out. But that doesn't mean it is impossible to understand it — in fact, everything that you need to know to be healthy using autophagy is actually pretty simple. Just like anything, there are specific methods to achieve autophagy at its full potential that will be explained throughout this book.

If you were just starting to explain autophagy to a friend, you might start out breaking down the word itself. You probably know that "auto" means "self," but you should also know that "phagy" means "eat." These are two roots from the Greek language, and together they create our English word. Autophagy occurs when our cells are put under a state of stress, and they eat parts of themselves that they no longer need or that even hinder the function of the cell.

The mitochondria is a prime example of this. The mitochondria is probably the most important organelle in your cell, and when your mitochondria aren't working the way it's supposed to, your cells will degrade their mitochondria and use them for raw material that your cells will use to build new mitochondria.

The mitochondria is not the only organelle that your cells do this for. All of your organelles are no longer useful after they degrade to a certain point, making it smarter for your cells to dispose of them and use the broken down parts to build new organelles. If they don't, organelles like damaged mitochondria would just be filling out more area in a cell than they deserve without actually serving a good purpose.

At times, you may think that I am overstating the importance of these microscopic processes in your body. However, these tiny events are far more important than you may realize. A mitochondria that is not well taken care of, whether from poor diet, lack of exercise, or lack of autophagy, can have deleterious effects on the body.

We have already talked at length about the relationship between low autophagy and neurodegenerative diseases, but it's important for you to know how big a part the mitochondria plays here.

A low-functioning mitochondria is closely linked to neurodegenerative diseases like Alzheimer's disease and Parkinson's disease. The best way to stave off a low-functioning mitochondria is by turning on autophagy.

It goes like this: you turn on autophagy through fasting, the keto diet, exercise, or a combination of these things; your cells build higher-functioning mitochondria to replace mitochondria that were taking a toll on the body; and finally, your healthier mitochondria runs the microscopic processes of your body smoothly and greatly reduces your risks of these neurodegenerative diseases. Of course, your mitochondria is not the only organelle that you have to think about, but it is the most important.

Sometimes the scientific terms can be overwhelming for anyone, so it is useful to think about autophagy in terms of an analogy. Whether you own a home or you rent a place, you probably have to deal with repairs someplace in your life. Even if you are on a lease for an apartment, you can deal with a broken vacuum cleaner or a broken dishwasher until someone from maintenance comes to fix it.

You don't have to know a lot about being handy to know one thing: it doesn't make sense to simply buy a new vacuum or dishwasher most of the time. Sometimes that may be the smartest course of action, but usually not. Usually, buying something new is too hasty. It saves you more money to try to fix the thing. You may have to end up buying something new, but it isn't smart at all to do that right away, knowing that you could potentially hold onto more money.

Your cells don't even have the choice to buy a new mitochondria, so they have to break down a bad one and use the parts to build a new one. They already have some supply of raw materials from broken down mitochondria if you turn on autophagy enough, so it is only logical for them to use them.

The cells throughout your body are quite resourceful. Autophagy occurs because they need to find a way to get food when they are not supplied with it. When this happens, they find nutrients in old things lying around that they don't need. That's where the discarded proteins, organelles, and toxins come in.

This process is the reason that humans can live for almost an entire month without eating. Your cells "eat" "themselves" (remember the origin of the word autophagy?), so for some period of time, they can go on without you eating food.

You may be surprised to hear that your system needs approximately 100 grams of protein on a daily basis. This is not an endorsement of a diet too high in protein, however, because you will be even more shocked by where the majority of the protein comes from: while approximately a fourth of it came out of eating throughout the day, the other three-fourths came out of autophagy.

That's right — most of the protein that cycles through your body doesn't even originate from the food you eat. It was already inside your body, and your cells naturally break it down for consumption. You might eat a slab of protein only once, but your cells eat that same protein multiple times over. It continuously cycles through your body in new forms.

It might start as a muscle cell; then, that cell's mitochondria is too dilapidated, so autophagy breaks it down and uses it as a new mitochondria. Later, that new mitochondria stops working efficiently, and autophagy turns it into a membrane.

The cells throughout your body can find protein nearly anywhere they go: in organelles, proteins that are no longer being used, and more. Without even your realizing it, your cells are building, destroying, and rebuilding these structures every day. Right now, somewhere in your body, one of your cells is constructing a new mitochondria with raw materials from a mitochondria it consumed during autophagy.

Any time your cells — or the cells of any plant or animal — go through a state of stress because of fasting or exercise, your cells start up autophagy. It is a cycle that is absolutely necessary for your survival as an organism. Without it, you could not keep on living.

I hope this chapter has provided you with a comprehensive but accessible resource to explain the biological mechanisms that make up autophagy. The rest of the book is dedicated to the lifestyle alterations you can make to turn your life around with autophagy. We will refer back to the science again from time to time, but only in reference to how to practically incorporate autophagy into your life.

Chapter 3
Why Intermittent Fasting

You have many things to choose from if you want to turn on autophagy throughout your body, but intermittent fasting is your best bet for several reasons. Methods like following the keto diet, exercising regularly and doing a full water fast work, but many people try these methods and give up on autophagy entirely because they can't commit to it in the long term.

IF (intermittent fasting) only requires you to restrict the eating you already do to a smaller window every day, and you still get to witness autophagy's anti-aging potential from this small change.

There is a serious risk of non-stop eating without taking a break by fasting. When you never fast, you are allowing the inevitable accumulation of toxins to damage your cells. This is why it is so important for you to turn on autophagy: so your cells can undo the damage that they endure from eating. Eating in itself takes a toll on your cells. The breakdown of food takes up energy. The particles that are not consumed simply take up space in your cells, making them less efficient.

Since it is hard for people to stick with regular water fasting without eventually dropping it completely, IF is the best way for most people to go. You can see the results that come from regular fasting, but you only have to make small changes, not big.

Do you remember what fundamental change in your body leads to autophagy? The answer is acute cellular stress. This stress can result from a variety of things, from starvation, exercise, and a sudden change from hot to cold or cold to hot. We haven't talked about the last one yet, but now is a good time to do so, because it provides a good illustration of why intermittent fasting is your best option.

You can actually turn on autophagy by simply stepping into a cold shower from room temperature — or vice versa, you could turn on autophagy by stepping into a very hot shower from room temperature, though I don't recommend it.

On a fundamental level, this works the same way as fasting and exercise because it puts your cells in a state of stress, just like when they are deprived of nutrients or when you give them microscopic tears to repair because of exercise. You could even step out of your house into the cold to turn on autophagy this way — or vice versa, step out of your room-temperature home into a scorching hot day.

Since this method of turning on autophagy fundamentally works the same as the ones we have discussed so far, why does it get so little attention? The reason is the same reason we are saving our discussion of water fasting for later.

Any method that achieves the result of autophagy is a valid method, but this book is not about turning on autophagy for a day. It is about turning it on basically every day so you can get the most benefit from it.

Some things seem interesting and exciting for a day or two, so much that you believe you will actually keep them up for longer. But then days pass, and you stop them completely. It is an issue of sustainability.

Ask yourself right now: are you truly going to step into a cold shower throughout the day to turn on autophagy? You might consider it plausible right now, but if you did it for a couple of days, you would realize that you are not going to keep it up. At least, it isn't likely that you will.

Intermittent fasting (IF), on the other hand, is a different story. Just don't eat anything from Noon to 8, for example. This is an easy example compared to some intermittent fasts, but the point being made is that not eating between the same times every day is infinitely more sustainable than stepping into a cold shower every day.

Beyond that, it is doubtful that a cold shower will have the same level of effect as intermittent fasting. There has been little if any, research on the effect of sudden temperature changes on autophagy, but it intuitively seems to have less of an effect from a purely subjective standpoint. You will feel your body go into shock for a moment, but it quickly passes. We can fairly safely deduce that autophagy is not as stimulated from this momentary change as it would from the bigger change over time that intermittent fasting introduces. However, a splash of cold water before getting out of the shower is known to have its own benefits, such as making you feel more awake.

It is also worthwhile to note that the cold shower method doesn't come with the health advantages that come from caloric restriction, as IF does. Study after study demonstrates that IF helps people who follow it keep up energy throughout the day; IF helps people burn body fat; IF even lowers the risk of heart disease and diabetes. Some of these effects may be linked to autophagy, which a cold shower would give you some of the benefits of.

However, you are far more likely to keep up a routine of eating less every day than you are to keep up a routine of stepping into a cold shower every day. You will also probably not see the same level of health benefit if you are stepping into cold showers but continuing to eat unhealthy foods.

Now, let's dive deeper into the mindset one must adopt if they want to keep up IF to turn on autophagy.

You can't start turning on autophagy with a mindset of stress, because it is not necessary for you to be stressed. It is only necessary for your cells to be stressed. Think about it this way: while you are sleeping, you aren't eating.

Technically speaking, from the standpoint of your cells, you are fasting while asleep. Your cells aren't getting any nutrients at this time, after all. While you are unconscious, you don't feel any stress at all, but your cells do. This is why people have the highest levels of autophagy while they are asleep. They feel some level of stress because they have no food to consume for seven to eight hours.

All the studies are telling us that fasting is the best way that we can turn on autophagy. The experts in nutrition and health are also telling us that intermittent fasting is the best way to go about fasting since it is the most sustainable. Compared to our example of the cold shower, you can see why this is the case.

Even though this is true, your best option for getting the most out of autophagy is still using several methods of autophagy stimulation at the same time. You should make IF your main method of doing this, but you will only get more benefit if you use other techniques as well.

The reason intermittent fasting turns on autophagy is because your cells need a constant stream of energy. Being microscopic, your cells can't store vast amounts of energy, and they have to constantly create new energy.

The cell stomach (lysosome) degrades the toxins it pulls in (in microautophagy) or that the autophagosome brings it (in macroautophagy), and then the cellular garbage is changed into raw materials that are later used to construct new cell parts.

What we have not yet touched on is the fact that the process of autophagy itself requires energy. In order to understand how energy works in a cell for the process of autophagy, and to understand how intermittent fasting won't leave you feeling tired, you need to understand ATP.

Many people are concerned about starting to do intermittent fasting because they incorrectly assume that eating less will deprive them of energy. On the contrary, scientists are telling us that people who fast have more energy than people who are constantly eating.

People who fast a lot in order to get a lot of autophagy have the most energy of all. This is because, as we have said, your cells themselves are constantly looking for sources of energy. Unlike you, they are not able to simply stop. They have a never-ending job to do. This means that even when you are not eating, they have to find more materials to break down for energy.

People who fast with IF have higher energy levels than people who don't because their cells are "cleaner." You see, people who don't fast may be feeding their cells with new nutrients constantly, but the constant stream of new food leads to vast amounts of waste in the cells.

The cells are not equipped to break down this waste when they are faced with a constant barrage of food. They have no reason to clean out their dead organelles, misfolded proteins, and the like when they are constantly provided with new food.

This is why people who fast have more energy. They may not be giving their cells new foods to eat, but their cells still have plenty to eat from the past. They have previous proteins to consume while waiting for you to eat again. Your cells have no choice but to do this constantly in order to survive.

And if this seems odd to you, don't forget that your cells are already doing it without being triggered directly with fasting. While you are sleeping, your cells still need energy to keep going, so they are breaking down their unused proteins, organelles, and foreign toxins during this time. Turning on autophagy during the day is no different; it is simply better for your body because you are going beyond the bare minimum autophagy that you get during sleep.

Since IF allows you to go through a good amount of autophagy every day, you don't have to worry about not getting enough of it. The cells in your body get a healthy amount of autophagy while you sleep, and during your fasting period during the day, they go the extra mile to break down the cellular garbage in your body even more.

We talked about caloric restriction earlier in the book. Don't forget that you are also getting this benefit from intermittent fasting. You will be able to start intermittent fasting with a positive mindset because you can be certain that you are doing something that is good for you. You also don't have to go through the stress of trying something more extreme like water fasting, because IF is far easier to start and to continue doing.

So many people try a water fast (consuming nothing but water for 24 hours or longer) and feel completely burned out of autophagy stimulation afterward. If you don't want this to happen to you, your best bet is to keep autophagy on as much as you can reasonably do it with IF.

Ultimately, the decision of how to turn on autophagy falls back on you. I recommend you consider your own health factors when you make this decision. For instance, if you have issues with your lungs or heart, you really shouldn't be considering a water fast at all. As good as the experience can be for your body and mind, you still have to think about your own biomarkers. A water fast does take a toll on people with any organs that cannot risk further trauma.

That's why I emphatically tell you now: if you are thinking of doing a water fast and you have had a previous issue with your lungs or heart, just don't do it. It is not worth the risk to these major organs. Besides, you can get nearly the same effect from regular intermittent fasting. There is no need for you to do a fast as intense as a water fast.

You should not start a child or teenager on intermittent fasting, either. This is because individuals in this age range are still going through a period of growth.

Theoretically speaking, anyone can get health benefits from turning on autophagy, but there is always a right and wrong context. This is an example of the wrong context for intermittent fasting.

You should also not do IF if you are a woman who is pregnant. Even if you have never had an issue with any of your major organs, your body is maintaining a delicate balance when you are carrying a child, and you can't disrupt that with IF.

Do not do IF if you have been diagnosed with diabetes. If you have diabetes, this should not come as a surprise. The amount of insulin in your body is too important to be tampered with through fasting, and IF isn't worth the risk in this case.

Finally, you should not start IF if you have ever been diagnosed with an eating disorder. Eating patterns are a difficult thing to change for anyone, but if you belong to this group, that may be especially true for you. There are cases of people with eating disorders who fell back into bad eating habits with the rationale that they are doing intermittent fasting. IF is meant to be a vehicle for good in your body, but if you use it as an excuse to fall out of doing good for your body, then it loses its entire purpose.

Truthfully, unless you have already gone to your general practitioner recently and they told you that you had no major health concerns, you should always talk to them before you make a major change in your eating patterns like starting IF. You want to be sure that your body can handle being deprived of nutrients for a set period every day.

IF may not be the most intense way to fast, but it is still a major change for your body, so you have to be careful with it. Only in the case that you are not a member of any of these groups should you proceed with IF.

Starting your First Intermittent Fast

We may have already gone into the mental aspect of the intermittent fast somewhat, but this is probably the most important aspect if you want to actually do it, so there is more for you to learn.

In specific, you need to learn this important lesson, a quote from Voltaire: "Perfect is the enemy of good." When this quote is applied to intermittent fasting and autophagy in general, it means that you can't be a perfectionist and do either of them well.

For example, if you want to do the intermittent fast and you completely forget about the fasting window and eat a snack, you might get frustrated and give up on IF completely. But in your first couple of weeks, you are bound to make lots of mistakes.

You are bound to eat during your fasting times. When this happens, you can't let it ruin the potential that autophagy could have in your life. It isn't the end of the world. You have to accept that you made a mistake and then keep going as if it didn't happen.

You are even bound to make mistakes after months of IF. No one is perfect. You may even do IF very well for months, get busy with a promotion in March, and fall out of intermittent fasting completely because of it. When that happens, you might feel tempted to give up on it too. You feel like you had a streak going, and you messed it up; it feels like you messed all of it up.

When it comes to intermittent fasting, you can't approach it with an all-or-nothing attitude. There will be weeks that everything goes exactly as you plan, and there will be weeks where it's as if you forgot everything you learned about autophagy. Remember: these blunders are inevitable. What will determine your success with IF and autophagy is your ability to get up and continue anyway.

There are lessons you can learn from your mistakes. If you keep eating during your fasting window in your initial week of IF, shorten your fasting window. You can always make it longer again later, but if you can't get yourself to fast for that long every day in the beginning, you can't let that stop you from fasting at all. Change your 12-hour intermittent fast to an 8-hour intermittent fast. Once you have a handle on the shorter fast, try to add a few more hours.

Perfect is the enemy of good. Perfectionism is the enemy of IF and autophagy.

We have a solid grasp of the mental aspect of IF now, so we can get more into the concrete details of what doing IF means.

You may be expecting there to be more to it than this, but besides everything else already included in this chapter, intermittent fasting involves exactly what the name suggests. You fast, but you don't fast continuously. You fast intermittently.

People who do IF first choose a number of hours that they want to fast every day. 8 hours is a decent place to start, but if this is too hard, you can go lower. Next, they pick a time during the day that this number of hours of fasting will go. For an 8-hour intermittent fast, you might choose not to eat between Noon and 8pm.

What happens next is easier said than done. You have to abstain from eating completely during this period of time in order to be faithful to your intermittent fast. If you can keep it up for a few weeks, you might want to extend the fast to 10, and eventually 12 hours. A 12-hour intermittent fast could mean eating breakfast at 8am, fasting until 9pm, and then eating dinner. Not everyone has to go this far, and not everyone has to go this far every day. What you decide to do is a matter of your own health situation and your own health goals.

Protein Cycling during Intermittent Fasting

It is time for you to learn about protein cycling. Protein cycling is a diet change that many people make when they do intermittent fasting. Basically, it means alternating between days of normal protein intake and low protein intake.

It is still important that you eat a normal amount of protein on the normal days because protein is an essential nutrient in your body. You need some level of normal protein every day, so your cells have it to build structures.

However, the low-protein days are important too. Having days where you consume little protein will further spur your cells to turn on autophagy during your fasting window. Your cells already have plenty of protein lying around as cellular garbage, so your cells can reliably use this as their source of protein on your low-protein days. (Don't forget the fact we learned earlier — your body processes 100 grams of it each day, and only a quarter of that comes from the food you eat!)

With all that in mind, you never want to consume lots of protein, no matter how important a nutrient it is. There is a very good reason for this. When you eat lots of protein, all you are doing is giving your cells lots of cellular garbage to clean out during autophagy. Your cells have to cycle between normal, non-stressed periods and autophagy periods, so it takes time for your cells to get rid of all of this excess.

When they take too long to do it, it eventually becomes toxic, as we have learned. Despite how essential a nutrient protein is, there is such thing as too much of a good thing, especially when it comes to protein.

When your diet is very high in protein, this hampers the progress of autophagy greatly. It does not hamper its progress as much as carbohydrates do, but it still slows things down. Instead of cleaning out your existing cellular garbage when you do IF, you will simply be cleaning out the junk left behind by all the protein you just ate.

Protein cycling gives us a great chance to discuss the importance of finding a balance between IF and a healthy diet. When you do protein cycling, you still need to eat the recommended amount of protein for a reason: it is an essential nutrient.

However, you can go too far in either direction. A lot of the foods people love contain protein, so it is common for people to eat far more protein than they should without even realizing it.

On the other hand, starving yourself of protein to the extreme is harmful, too. If you do this, you may experience loss in muscle tone that is usually associated with fasts more extreme than intermittent fasting.

To do protein cycling right, simply eat the recommended amount of protein every other day, and half or less that amount on your other days.

This is not only about protein, though. Even though IF is a fast meant for everyone, there are still ways we can take it too far. Take someone who makes their fasting window too long: let's say, 14 hours. That would mean they eat for an hour in the morning and then eat again for an hour before bed. This is absolutely unhealthy, and I recommend not doing this. It is still necessary for the body to receive some nutrients, even when fasting.

I especially advise against it because the IF is meant to be done every day. If you are fasting for 14 hours every day, that could have serious consequences on your body. With a water fast, you may fast for as much as 24 or 48 hours, but the difference is the frequency. Someone can do a water fast all day on Sunday and then go back to their normal eating patterns on Monday.

But if they do IF for 14 hours a day, there is never a time they return to their regular eating pattern. Their regular eating pattern involves consuming far too infrequently.

Maybe you are familiar with the concept of yin and yang from Taoism. The yang gives, and the yin takes. To find a balance between a healthy diet and IF, keep thinking of eating as yang and IF as yin. You need yang to fill yourself up with fresh nutrients.

When you are following IF, you do this outside of your fasting window. You need yin to cleanse your cells of the toxins produced from yang.

Too much of yang (eating) and too much of yin (fasting) both have negative consequences. The key is to find a balance between the two; this will allow you to get the benefits of both.

Put another way, don't let yourself believe that "extra" fasting will lead too better health outcomes. It won't. If you truly want to be healthy, you need to find the right about eating for your yang and the right amount of fasting for your yin.

Chapter 4
Keto Diet

Intermittent fasting alone will help you get rid of body fat, improve the quality of your epidermis (your skin), and change the way you think about eating. However, you can get the most out of IF by combining it with the keto diet. Keto and IF are a perfect match. The main characteristic of keto is drastically reducing your carb consumption, and this would also be a help to your body to start autophagy because carbs take a long time to break down.

If your main goal is to lose weight, keto and IF will also work together to help achieve this goal. Autophagy helps in this regard by cleaning toxins from your body, while the keto diet puts your body into ketosis, creating chemicals called ketones that aid in burning fat.

There is a good number of people who follow the keto diet but don't even know what autophagy is. This is a real shame because the two can work wonderfully together. While turning on autophagy is one of the best things you can do for your overall health, the truth is that a lot of people start following the keto diet for the sole purpose of losing weight. If your main goal with autophagy is to lose weight, then the ketogenic diet may be your new best friend.

You will have a lot of changes in your body if you follow a lifestyle of both turning on autophagy and following the keto diet, though, so keep that in mind. You can't expect to make such drastic changes without running into some things that you didn't expect. Both things have in common that people tend to feel slightly low on energy at first, but end up feeling more energetic once all the health benefits start to kick in.

All in all, autophagy is not something that can be reduced to a tool for losing weight, whereas the ketogenic diet can be, more or less. The entire purpose of keto is to deprive the body of carbs, causing it to release ketones that will then help you burn fat.

On the other hand, autophagy usually helps people lose weight because the means of turning on autophagy result in losing weight. Autophagy itself is about maintaining a well-balanced body, but fasting, dieting, and exercising are all the means of turning on autophagy, and all of those things also help you lose weight.

Changing your diet, in particular, will help you lose weight. When people learn how much exercise it takes to burn 100 calories, they tend to be very surprised. While exercise is an important part of the process for losing weight if you are already overweight, no matter your size, diet is always the most important. People who lose weight do it because they stop consuming more calories than they burn off with exercise.

The keto diet follows this rule, too. Being a change in the content of what you eat, it will ultimately be more effective than anything else. It also comes with the activation of ketosis, which is part of what makes it so popular.

Not only does keto involve eating foods that will keep you from putting on so much weight, but the lack of carbs will lead to a chemical process that helps you burn the fat you already have. Combined with autophagy-stimulating methods like exercise and intermittent fasting, you can't go wrong with using keto to lose weight.

Besides all the reasons I've already listed, I recommend doing intermittent fasting alongside the keto diet for one reason in particular. There are a lot of common mistakes people make when they decide to do intermittent fasting, and perhaps the most common one is not thinking about their diet when they are not fasting.

You could be entirely faithful to your 10-hour IF, but then choose to eat foods full of saturated fats and carbohydrates when you are not within your fasting window. I want to be very clear on this now: if you don't eat healthy when you aren't fasting, you really shouldn't be fasting in the first place, because you are wasting your time.

Diet truly is everything when it comes to health — or as the cliché goes, "You are what you eat."

If you are keeping up a sedentary lifestyle, eating foods loaded with sugar, salt, saturated fats, and carbs, and keeping habits like smoking or alcohol abuse, you might as well not fast in the first place, because it isn't doing what it should be doing for you.

At that point, you are using it as an excuse not to be healthy in other aspects of your life. If you keep up habits like these — habits that everyone knows are bad for your body — doing intermittent fasting isn't going to reverse all of those consequences for you.

This is where keto comes in. It gives you a template to follow for the food you eat when you aren't on the fast; that way, you are responsible for that aspect of your health as well. It will prevent you from running into this common mistake of thinking IF will cover for all your other poor health choices. And at the same time, you will get to enjoy all the other positive components we talked about.

In other words, following a keto diet while you do intermittent fasting is your best bet for keeping on track with your health overall instead of using it as an excuse to be unhealthy outside of your fast. You may not be ready to change your eating patterns to the keto diet at the beginning of your IF, but you can use this chapter as a guide for when you do.

Did you know that the median person living in the United States gets half of their calories from carbs? This country is also known as the one with the highest number of overweight and obese people — it can't be a coincidence that the health of their diet is one specific nutrient.

The keto diet combats this pattern of eating tons of carbs. If you follow keto, you don't eat more than 30 grams of it a day. As an added bonus, you keep your cholesterol low and eat unsaturated fats, both of which are good things for efficient autophagy.

Sometimes it's hard to remember something entirely without a vivid illustration from an example, so consider this: if you follow a diet low in carbs like the keto diet, your body will be finished digesting your food and start the process of autophagy in four hours. Alternatively, if you eat too many carbs, you slow down this process significantly. Your system will now take 8 hours to digest your food; 8 hours to begin autophagy.

Don't misunderstand: when you fast for 8 hours after eating, in reality, you are fasting for 4. And that's assuming you ate a meal low in carbs. Your body doesn't go through autophagy while you are digesting, and carbs take a long time to digest. If you didn't see how keto and IF were so complementary before, you must see it now.

In the next section, we'll go more in-depth on the mechanics of the ketogenic diet. After that, we'll give you plenty of advice on how to follow through with it.

The Mechanisms of Keto

Here, you will learn why keto is so helpful as an aide to making the rate of autophagy go up. At the end of the day, what you choose to eat and what you choose to do with your body are your choices alone, but I hope that we succeed in convincing you of coupling your IF with keto.

When the body breaks down glucose (the natural sugar from food), it uses carbs. The keto diet takes advantage of this and causes your system to produce ketones to replace carbs when you stop consuming as much carbs. Your body still needs to break down the glucose, so you are basically forcing it to do it by producing a lot more of a chemical that will help you burn body fat.

People who are on the keto diet are doing it as a means to the end of activating ketosis in their bodies. They do this by eating a far higher proportion of healthy fats than carbs. Since your body will always burn carbs before it burns anything else, depriving it of this chemical sends your body in ketosis, giving you a lot of ketones in your bloodstream.

You have probably thought for a long time that you need to watch out for fat above all else, but this is misinformation. It is not the amount of fat that you eat, but the kinds of fat that matters.

What happens for most people who find themselves putting on weight is that (1) they consume a lot of carbs, (2) their bodies burn through the carbs over a long period, and (3) their bodies leave behind tons of fat because they were so preoccupied with the carbs. Therefore, turning on ketosis has the twofold benefit of unleashing ketones to burn fat and to tell your system to focus on burning fat instead of spending all of its time on carbs.

Autophagy is more potent when you are on the keto diet because it is a diet consisting of few carbs and many healthy fats. Healthy fats are necessary for all parts of your body to perform their tasks, while carbs are substance that will slow down autophagy the most the more of it that you consume. Keto keeps you from eating foods that would seriously hinder the effectiveness of your autophagy, while also eating healthy, unsaturated fats that your cells can use to build new structures.

You can think of autophagy and keto as strongly linked using an analogy: intermittent fasting is to autophagy as the keto diet is to ketosis.

You use the first to turn on the second. You use fasting to turn on autophagy, while you use the keto diet to turn on ketosis. Ketosis is the central process and goal of the keto diet wherein your body produces the ketones that will greatly help to burn through your body fat.

We have already gone over the effects of autophagy and ketosis that you will feel, see in the mirror, and experience by living a life feeling healthier and living longer. However, you might be curious if there is a way you can measure your level of autophagy or ketosis in a more objective way.

While it does require some commitment, there is a way you can do this using the glucose-ketone index. Looking at this index will give you a pretty good indication of whether you are going through autophagy and ketosis (with this measurement, the two almost always go hand in hand). The first thing you have to do is purchase a blood sugar tester.

When you take a sample of your blood, be sure to do it when you are currently fasting. If you don't, you won't get a precise reading. This is because your body has a significant amount of glucose when you are not fasting, and the blood sugar levels that you read won't tell you anything about your autophagy.

First, you need to know the formula for the glucose-ketone index. When you draw blood for the blood sugar meter, you will see the glucose value and the ketone value. Before you do anything, divide glucose by 18; however, only do this if your blood sugar meter uses mmol/L. When the meter uses mg/dL, you don't divide by 18 or do anything. Then, you have to divide your glucose value by the ketone value. Finally, take this number and divide it by 3.4. Then you will have your glucose-ketone index.

You don't want your glucose-ketone index to be below 3. This is a level at which people have seizures or may be suffering from cancer. An index from 3 to 6 is usually a sign that you are obese or have diabetes. This is not a desirable glucose-ketone index either.

Finally, we have an index between 6 and 9. This is what you want as someone who is aiming for autophagy and ketosis. A person between 6 and 9 can easily lose weight or keep at the weight they are at. Finally, an index above 9 means you are not looking at a level of autophagy or ketosis that is sufficient.

Even though the index seems completely flawless and objective since it comes from numbers on a blood test, you need to take it with a grain of salt. A glucose-ketone index slightly below 6 doesn't definitely mean that you are obese, for instance. These numbers fluctuate somewhat, just like your weight. By the same token, having an index from 6 to 9 is not a sure way of saying you are the portrait of perfect health.

There are a lot of things that affect the level of your blood sugar, so an index like this is not completely dependable. You can't even know for sure if your index is where it is because of keto or intermittent fasting. Always use several indicators to decide if you are generally healthy. Ask yourself questions like: have I been losing or gaining weight? Does my skin look dry? How do I feel subjectively? That third question could seem to have less of an impact than the others, but you will be surprised how good you feel compared to before once you incorporate keto and IF into your daily routine. You have to pay attention to subjective experiences as well because your quality of life matters a great deal.

It should go without saying, but just to be clear, you always have to use more than one measure to assess your health. Continue to go to the doctor and be honest with them at all times. Listen to them and be open to what they say.

With all these caveats aside, the glucose-ketone index is a pretty solid way of figuring out if you are meeting your goals in ketosis and autophagy. You are probably in good shape as far as keto and autophagy if you are between 3 and 9.

Keto: The Practical Walkthrough

Before you get into this intermittent fasting and keto business, you are going to want to know what you should expect. Let's go over what happens over time for someone who does IF and follows the keto diet when not in the fasting window.

When twelve hours pass that you are on the keto diet, you already start the initial stages of ketosis. You are already burning through body fat without even working for it with exercise. As an extra perk, some of the fat that you burn through is converted into more ketones in the liver to burn fat.

By now, your body is relying on ketones for energy instead of glucose. This is yet another boon for autophagy since any significant level of glucose will stop significant autophagy in its tracks.

You will even feel a difference in how you think and feel. This is because your brain cells are using ketones for energy as well. There is a very good chance you will feel more clear-headed when your body is in this state of ketosis and autophagy. As a result, you may find yourself in a better mood.

Though the keto side of things is more about losing weight than overall health, you will be pleased to know that ketones don't create nearly as much inflammation as glucose does, either. For people who are trying to lose weight, inflammation tends to be high on the list of health concerns, so this is just another reason to do keto.

Let's fast-forward to 18 hours into IF and keto. You are now at a level of fat-burning and ketone-producing that you have not reached before. The amount of ketones in your body is much more than, probably, ever in your entire life.

When 24 hours pass on IF and keto, autophagy is seeing its best days. Since your system is running so smoothly because of the ketones, your cells are working tirelessly to dispose of waste materials, convert them into raw materials in autophagy, and then turn them into useful structures in the cell cycle.

48 hours into IF and keto, your ketosis is at its highest level. Autophagy peaks near 24 hours, while keto does around this point. Because of this, your growth hormones start reaching very high levels. Growth hormones have many benefits, including keeping fat tissue from building up and reducing muscle loss that comes with age.

Though we have already reached the acumen of performance from IF and keto, they still both do great work if you continue following them past the 48-hour mark. At 54 hours of keto and IF, your insulin is at its lowest level yet.

Keeping a low insulin is a great health goal to have because doing so hinders mTOR, a gene that stops autophagy from turning on when activated. As an added benefit, low insulin tends to go together with low inflammation.

Finally, after three days, or 72 hours of IF and keto, your cells are getting rid of poorly performing immune cells, and they make new immune cells to replace them. Having young immune cells may indeed be one of the greatest non-cosmetic consequences of doing IF and the keto diet together.

So as not to mislead you, I will reiterate: the ketogenic diet is in no way required to turn on autophagy in your body. However, as you can see from this progression over 72 hours, the two lifestyle changes complement each other perfectly. It is almost like they were meant to be done together.

When you do IF with keto, the high level of unsaturated fats will cause you to go through even more autophagy than you would have otherwise. When you lose weight from these lifestyle changes, you won't have to deal nearly as much with the pesky issue of loose skin, because while keto burns your fat, autophagy will restore your skin cells after they move because of weight loss.

If you read all of this and still decide to do IF without following the keto diet, at least make sure you keep a low-carb diet. Remember: autophagy does not actually start significantly until you are done digesting your food, and when you eat more than a low amount of carbs, they take about 8 hours to digest. This is 4 more hours that your cells will not be going through autophagy.

While I have been going over all the good things about keto so far, there are certain warnings for you to keep in mind. For one, doctors warn that consuming a lot of fats — even healthy fats — can lead to damage to your gut.

This is not to say to avoid fats altogether, because you need them. However, you can overdo anything, and healthy, unsaturated fats is one of them.

Originally, the ketogenic diet was conceived of as a treatment for people with epilepsy. Patients with epilepsy who tried this diet had half as many seizures as a result. Amazingly, they did not even see the seizures return when they stopped following keto.

The key to doing keto in a healthy way is the same as doing anything healthily: moderation. Despite what you may hear, it is not a good idea to follow a keto diet all of the time, no matter how badly you want to lose weight. Even epilepsy patients don't follow keto all of the time — what does that tell you?

Just stick with the original formula for keto: consume a lot of healthy fats, a not-low not-high level of protein, and a low level of carbs. Note that you shouldn't eat no carbs, because you do need them. You just don't need so much of them all the time. If you're feeling sick because of keto, that's a good sign that you should take a break from it, and wait to try again until you feel better.

Following the original formula for keto gives you sufficient protein for your cells to build new structures and sufficient calories to have enough energy. Traditionally, you follow a ratio of 4:1 of fat to protein and carbs. However, most experts agree that 3:1 is just fine. The best way to achieve this ratio is by avoiding starchy foods, breads, pastas, and grains, and sugars. You can still eat foods like nuts and some dairy products.

To follow the keto diet, the healthy way, listen to the following advice, and heed it. If you did keto for the past two weeks, you should be thinking about going back to a typical proportion of carbohydrates in your diet for a while.

It definitely isn't good for you to go without a normal amount of carbs for an extended period of time. It's just the same as I always say in this book: going too far stops being good, and starts being bad.

Just like people can take intermittent fasting too far sometimes, there are perhaps more people who take keto too far. Unfortunately, when we want to lose weight, we lose ourselves in that goal sometimes and start doing things that we know are bad for us. As an author concerned for your general health, you should know that I want you to think of your weight only as one part of the picture of your health. Losing weight is part of the picture of getting healthier, but not by any means. It is totally counterproductive to do unhealthy behaviors in order to lose weight.

To close, you want to make sure to stick the most important things about keto in your mind so you can make an intelligent decision about whether you will start following it. If you follow keto, you will start replacing the high volume of carbs that you eat with more healthy fats. You can think of "healthy" fats as synonymous with "unsaturated" fats.

Practically speaking, this means you have to stay away from the bottom of the food pyramid as much as possible: that's breads, grains, and pastas. It means avoiding beans, sugars, and snack foods, as these products are notoriously anti-keto.

By following this eating pattern, you will start ketosis in your body, since your system can't rely on glucose for energy anymore. It will start relying on ketones from your liver, a chemical that will greatly aid in burning fat.

Finally, the warning to remember with keto is not to let ketosis go on for too long. Two weeks is about the time that you need to start thinking about going back to non-keto foods for a while. But as long as you keep that in mind, you can harness the power of keto and intermittent fasting to lose weight and keep your body detoxified.

Chapter 5
Extended Water Fasting

Once you get into the habit of intermittent fasting, you might get more curious about more intense fasts like the water fast. You need to be mindful of what your body can handle with any kind of fast, but this is particularly true with extended water fasting because you will deprive your body of nutrients for as long as 48 hours at a time if you choose so. This chapter will tell you how to do your first water fast in a safe way, approaching it from both the physical and psychological perspective.

Your first-ever fast doesn't have to be a water fast, but I highly recommend that you try to do one at least once. You don't only do it for the physical benefits to your body; you also do it for the way it changes your mind.

When you go even 24 hours without eating in today's culture in which we never stop eating, it makes you see things differently. You start looking at food in a new way. You may even see things beyond food in a new way, too. Much like what happens when you do a keto diet for a long time, if you do a water fast, you are likely to experience a refreshing clear-headedness unlike you ever have before.

You might have run into the phrase "dry fasting" before, and while we're on the topic of these intense fasts, you should know this: it is completely fine for most people to go with only water and no food for 24 or even 48 hours.

But not only is going without water for this long bad for you (as in a "dry fast"), there is no reason for it. Drinking water does not stop autophagy the way that eating food does. If you did a dry fast, you would be dehydrating yourself for no reason at all.

A number of religious traditions include fasting for a reason. No religion is really centered on the health of the body; the reasons for fasting in these cases are usually for a renewal of spirit and mind. Whether you abide by the rest of the traditions of any particular religion, you can feel confident that there must be something to a pure water fast if people have been doing it for hundreds or thousands of years.

Like with intermittent fasting, there isn't much to say about water fasting as far as explaining what you have to do to water fast. If you consume nothing but water for 24 hours, you have done a water fast. However, there's still plenty more than that for you to keep in mind before you embark on such a feat.

First, you might wonder what the point of this intense of a fast is. Do you not get as much health benefit from a regular intermittent fasting routine? The simple answer is technically, no, you don't. While anyone can get more than what they need from IF, water fasting is for those who want to go that extra mile.

Consider this. If you are in the middle of your fasting window for your 8-hour intermittent fast and you eat a granola bar, you miss out on all of the benefits you would have gleaned from autophagy. That's because eating anything at all brings your blood sugar up, turning autophagy off. It may seem strange that even eating 70 calories would throw off autophagy so much, but it's how this biological process works.

Where does water fasting come in? You can get a decently potent autophagy process going if you are faithful to your intermittent fast, and you abstain from eating for a full eight hours. Earlier, we learned that assuming you follow a low-carb diet, you are still digesting your food for four hours after eating. That makes an eight-hour fast a "true" four-hour fast.

This is not to discredit the shorter fasts whatsoever. After all, your body's natural autophagy happens while you are sleeping, and assuming you don't eat four hours before bed, that's still "only" eight hours of autophagy. Combined with four extra hours of autophagy during the day, you are still going to extra mile to detox your cells and keep them healthy.

However, you might see the appeal of a water fast after seeing it this way. A water fast isn't something you do every day, of course, and not even every week, for most people who do them. Most people who do water fasting do it a handful of times every month so they can get as full an experience of autophagy for their bodies. Without water fasting, you can't truly achieve this level of autophagy. Most days, you have to eat, and after sleep, there are only so many hours in the day that you can turn on a high level of autophagy through fasting.

Occasional water fasts are an option for people who want to satisfy their desire to do a deep cleanse of their cellular waste. They continue to do intermittent fasting every day so they can get a regular cleanse, but every other week or so, they choose to do a water fast and truly get as much out of autophagy as can be gotten.

Don't make the mistake many people make with water fasting and drink coffee. For some reason, there seems to be this idea that you can drink coffee while water fasting. This is not true. Coffee breaks a fast. If you are doing a water fast, you can't drink juice, coffee, tea, or any drink with a substance that your body would have to process. The processing of that substance will cause autophagy to cease, completely ruining the whole point of water fasting.

There are writers on the subject of water fasting who concede that these drinks will stymie autophagy to some extent, but they say that at the end of the day, it doesn't make much of a difference. I beg to differ. We have a lot of scientific evidence of the effectiveness of pure water fasting — we don't have any evidence to back up a pure water fast, minus some coffee here and there.

Even a cup of coffee at the beginning of your fast can mess things up. Don't take the risk when you are already looking to get as much as possible out of autophagy.

Another common mistake is consuming flavored water during the water fast. Do not do this — again, the flavoring has something that your body has to break down. When your body breaks down chemicals, autophagy stops. You should even stay away from smells of flavor. It sounds bizarre, but even the smell of real or artificial food causes a parasympathetic reaction from your vagus nerve.

This reaction will actually keep autophagy from happening to a significant degree because it stimulates mTOR, a gene that will stop autophagy when activated. It may feel like there is such a delicate balance, but if you are water fasting to maximize the potential of autophagy, these are the things you have to consider.

Don't even take vitamins or supplements that purport to boost autophagy during your water fast. Not to beat a dead horse, but your body has to process that, and then autophagy won't start until it's done.

People who advocate for these supplements say that supplements don't have enough digestible chemicals to stop autophagy from happening, but they don't really know this is the case. They are just selling a supplement. (On a side note, there is no official supplement that is known to turn on or even aid autophagy at this moment, so you shouldn't bother shopping around for them.)

We went over what happens hour by hour when you combine IF with the keto diet. What happens over time when you start a water fast?

You will be happy to learn that in your neurons, the autophagosomes increase significantly after just 12 hours of fasting. Remember that this isn't really because of the "water fast," but because going much further than this length of time starts to be impossible for an IF practitioner, simply because of a lack of hours in the day.

The great thing about this is if you choose to make your IF fasting window include the evening right before you go to bed, and you rest well that night, you can still get to this 12-hour mark without even water fasting. Your brain should be feeling refreshed in the morning because of the deep autophagy activity its cells went through.

I hope I have sold you on water fasting, or at least got you interested on trying it later. Our next section will tackle the things you can expect during a water fast and how to prepare to do one.

Water Fasting: a Practical Walkthrough

Before we begin, keep in mind that the water fast is not meant for people inexperienced in fasts of any kind. If this book was the first thing to make you think about fasting, you should get used to regular intermittent fasting before you try this. A water fast under 48 hours is perfectly safe, but my reasoning is that you might get burnt out of autophagy completely if you fail to meet your own standards in the water fast, and we want to avoid that.

That said, it's ultimately your choice what you will do. Perhaps you read our introduction to the concept, and you are already all-in on this experience. In that case, make sure you read carefully and always think of safety and health first.

You should take a guess about what people usually notice first as a consequence of water fasting. It's an easy one, so don't overthink it.

If you guessed that they lost weight, you would be right. It shouldn't really be surprising that refraining from eating for an extended period of time causes people to lose weight. This shows that at the end of the day, losing weight is a matter of not eating so many calories without a plan to burn them off.

Your body relies on glucagon (glucose) after only a day of water fasting. You run through all the glucagon in your liver from just water fasting for 24 hours. When that happens, your system uses protein and fat for energy.

It is similar to how the keto diet causes you to start running on ketones, but instead of ketones, you burn through the protein and fat. This is yet another reason not to bring too much protein into your system — your system might choose to burn through protein instead of fat, which is definitely not a desired outcome.

Because of this, your weight drops very quickly. In only two days of water fasting, you lose up to two pounds every day.

This might make you feel tempted to water fast for long periods of time. There are certainly people who go longer than a day or two, and you can join them if you would like, given that you think you are ready. However, there has been some research about the impact of water fasting on autophagy, and scientists suggest that the number of autophagosomes in your cells caps around 36 hours of water fasting.

Now, if you water fast for longer than that, you are still going through autophagy for longer. Therefore, you are still getting this out of it. But in most cases and for most people, 36 to 48 hours will be your maximum for water fasting. Don't lose sight of the fact that you ultimately want to turn on autophagy for your general health. You are fasting for this purpose, not to just drop as many pounds as possible. The goal you set means everything for your health.

As someone who has done countless water fasts and remembers their early ones vividly, you need to keep in mind that the first day is the hardest. This is because it is very easy to spend the whole time thinking about food and what you want to eat. A sudden rush of cravings is very common for people on their first day.

When you last through the first day, however, you will stop having such strong cravings. They no longer have such a hold over you. Losing cravings is a really big part of water fasting because when you have them, they essentially give you the feeling of being hungry when you do not actually need food — you are just craving it. People are not good at telling the difference between the two. Once the cravings are gone, your health, in the long run, is positively affected, because you stop feeling "hungry" for these foods, you were merely craving all along.

Be cautious about the addiction to weight loss. Some people who get into water fasting, or even fasting in general, start having unhealthy habits once they realize how much weight they can lose.

But we have already gone over the dangers of pairing fasting with eating disorders. This time, I'm talking about the danger of inconsistency. Some people will do a water fast until they are happy with the number of pounds they lost, and then they go back to their normal life of consuming lots of carbs, not exercising, and so on.

You have to make fasting a normal part of your life if you want it to change your life. Too many people think they can exercise or fast a couple times a year and think it will make a difference.

Consistency is everything with autophagy. You can glean serious benefit from it if you water fast a few times a month, or intermittent fast every day consistently. You don't see any benefit from just doing it whenever you feel like it and completely forgetting about it the rest of the time.

We are almost done with the physical side of water fasting; then, we can get to the psychological side.

A large part of the purpose of the water fast is a detox. Since a water fast is so intense, you see intense health benefits from it. However, your senses are pretty attuned from the food deprivation while your body simultaneously goes through these shifts. One such shift is when you feel autophagy burning through your fat.

It is not a sharp pain like a knife, but it is far from comfortable, and you should be ready for it. Since it means fat is leaving your body, you are probably more than happy to feel this discomfort. Still, it's good to be aware of it, so you aren't surprised. You had tons of toxins inside your fats, and now they are all being released at the same time. You can't expect to leave them behind without this discomfort.

Losing the weight itself can also be uncomfortable. You may get a weird feeling in your skin. Be aware that these feelings are perfectly normal, but still be aware of the difference between this and being sick. If you do not go to dangerous extremes in your water fast, you shouldn't have to worry about this at all.

We have discussed the danger of water fasting when you have an eating disorder, but take what I am about to tell you with the knowledge that this is about something else. Sometimes, when people do a water fast for a while, they enjoy the high they get from it so much that they keep chasing after that high as if it is a drug.

Like I said, this is different from fasting for too long to lose weight. Here, I am talking about someone chasing a drug-like high that they get from fasting. This is something to watch out for, too. They keep fasting for longer and longer because the last fasting high didn't satisfy them.

Don't do water fasting if you are doing it for a high. Do it for the physical and psychological benefits. After reading the coming section about the psychology of the water fast, it will be easier to get your mind in the right place and make sure you are water fasting for the right reasons.

Finally, it's time for the technicalities of how you can get the water fast right. Although you can't consume anything with calories during this fast, everyone needs electrolytes in their body every day, and you might not have them in your water at home. For your health and safety, it's important that you still get electrolytes on your days doing a water fast.

There are a few ways to go about getting electrolytes. You can consume supplements with electrolytes with your water. However, the easier thing to do is just drinking water with a sprinkle of salt and a lemon to make sure it has electrolytes.

Next, there is the matter of what you put in your body when the water fast is over. There is definitely a right and a wrong way to break a water fast. The absolute wrong way to do it would be eating a plate full of bread when it is over. This would overwhelm your body with carbs to digest after making it accustomed to nothing at all for the length of the fast.

If you eat a lot of carbs to break a water fast, your blood will get a surge of insulin to break down the carbohydrates. Insulin requires a good amount of electrolytes, and while you should have electrolytes in your system, you definitely won't have a sufficient amount for the undertaking of digesting a bunch of carbs.

There is real physical danger to breaking a water fast this way. Doing so can lead to high blood pressure, a heart attack, and even sudden death. Thankfully, it is not hard to do things the right way.

If your first meal has to have carbs, make sure it's low carbs. But before you break the fast at all, make sure to get a thymine supplement into your system, as well as B vitamins.

The general rule of thumb for the meal that breaks your fast is 10 calories for every kilogram of your mass. You shouldn't eat a big meal, to begin with. Slowly introduce small, healthy snacks into your system. Also, be sure to have lots of water during this time, still using supplements or lemon and salt for electrolytes. It is good to introduce some healthy juice to your body at this time — all-natural, nothing with artificial preservatives.

Inside the Mind of a Person doing a Water Fast

The key to success and safety with the water fast is going into it with your goals clearly defined. Ask yourself right now, since you are pretty far into the book at this point: what are you doing this for? Do you want to lose weight? Do you want to look younger? Do you want to live longer?

While it's true that autophagy achieves all three for you, you still need to have a purpose for autophagy that is for you and you alone. If you don't, you won't be very likely to change entire aspects of your lifestyle for it. Once you have a well-defined purpose for something, all the rest starts to fall into place, because you know what you want to do.

The opposite of that is when you don't have a well-defined purpose at all, and you give up easily. If you don't know why you're doing something, it is very easy for you to give up on it. You don't even have a point in continuing with it, so why wouldn't you?

It is very easy to start things. Anyone can start a 300-word novel. Anyone can start a sculpture. What makes you accomplished is when you can start something and finish it. Autophagy and water fasting is no different. If you have a clear reason you want to see through your first water fast to the end, you will be far less likely to fall out of it.

Having your goal in mind isn't just a preventive measure against giving up; it's almost a way for you to do things the right way. If you are in the middle of a water fast, you might be tempted to get a snack, even though you know it ruins the purpose of the entire fast. When you already know your goal for water fasting, though, you are a lot less likely to fall for temptations like these.

You can tell yourself, "I am fasting to lose weight. I won't lose weight if I add more food into my stomach during this fast, so I'm not going to cheat on the fast with that cookie."

Alternatively, if you went into your water fast without a goal like this, things would probably go a lot different. You would see the cookie and say, "Well, it is my first-day fasting. I can do things the correct way next time." Since you don't have a clear reason for water fasting, there just isn't that emotional weight to cheating on the fast that there otherwise would be.

A second crucial but often overlooked part of the mindset of someone who succeeds in the water fast is knowledge of fasts and autophagy. Plenty of people believe they know things about these topics, so much that they actually do fasting the way they believe is correct, whether it is right or not.

Fortunately, you have this whole book of easy-to-understand information about fasting and autophagy. You could return to it if you need to know more, but chances are, you are absorbing it so well that it isn't even necessary. You already have this second crucial part of the mindset covered.

Finally, there is the third and last part of the mindset required to succeed in a water fast, and it is adaptability. You have lots of goals that propelled you to do a water fast in the first place, but the one that will carry the fate of all the others is your adaptability to a new, healthier way of living. This mental aspect will determine if you continue water fasting a few times a month, or if it is just something you do one time and never again.

You will get some health benefits from the autophagy that comes from water fasting one time, but these benefits are pointless if you don't keep it up. That's why it's so crucial that you adapt well to the new habits you formed and do it again in a few weeks.

Chapter 6
Metabolic Autophagy Foods

You can find many writers who will sell you supplements claiming to boost autophagy. While the ingredients in these supplements may be what you are looking for, there is one crucial thing to know: getting these nutrients from supplements will not have the same benefit as from consuming them in your food.

The famous omega-3 fats from fish are a prime example. There is an overwhelming amount of evidence to suggest the great benefit of getting these healthy fats from fish, but none to suggest you will get the same reward by getting them from a supplement. To save your wallet and your health, this chapter will walk you through many tips like this so you can eat the right foods while using techniques to turn on autophagy.

There are always people out there trying to tell you there is an easy way of doing things. I am not here to tell you that turning on autophagy has to be hard, because it doesn't. But any time someone tells you that you can make autophagy happen by taking a supplement that they are selling you, you can know that their agenda is to sell their product, not to tell you the truth about autophagy.

That said, pharmacists are working on such a product. We are not there yet, though, and anyone claiming that we are is lying.

People are always going to be resistant to doing things the slow way. We are always looking for shortcuts so we don't have to put in the time or effort. There rarely is a true, easy way — however, that doesn't mean it has to be complicated. Turning on autophagy is simple, but not easy.

After all, you only have to eat the right foods, fast at some level, get plenty of sleep, and exercise. It's not as if these concepts are hard to understand; it is just that action is always harder than talk. Any time someone tells you that you can turn on autophagy without doing these things is not telling the truth. This could be true in the future, but we are not there yet.

These truths may be a bit hard to swallow at first, but as you get into the right habits that turn on autophagy, you will realize that it is completely true when I say this stuff is simple, but not easy.

With all that in mind, you are ready to learn about what you should eat to get the most out of your autophagy.

Eating Right for Autophagy

It is totally understandable to be overwhelmed by this information at first, so don't be shy about reading through it for mere familiarity at first. This is information that you would be best off referring back to when you need it.

The most basic principle of eating right for autophagy is making sure you are getting significant autophagy in every organ in your body. So far, we have only talked about autophagy in terms of cells, but that is not what our goal is at the end of the day. We want the autophagy to aim for the betterment of our heart, liver, and lungs most of all. There are foods that will help autophagy target these organs, and we are about to go over them.

While there are no supplements that turn on autophagy directly, there are supplements that help you target the betterment of these vital organs. However, they are only effective if they are combined with a full of nutrients and vitamins. In other words, there is no point in taking a bunch of supplements if you are not eating healthy as well. It is no different from when we said you can't expect to fast to turn on autophagy and have it counteract all the other unhealthy habits you might have like drinking heavily, smoking, overeating, and so forth. The principle of consistency in autophagy requires that you keep a regular schedule of autophagy stimulating habits while also being healthy in other aspects at the same time.

You learned a bit about healthy fats in our chapter about the ketogenic diet, but there is still more for you to learn. Omega-3 fats are an important fat for you to get, but like we said, there is no evidence that you will get the same benefit from it if you are only taking supplements that give you Omega-3 fats — and on the other side of things, there is plenty of evidence that getting Omega-3 fats from actual food has lots of benefits.

This idea applies to supplements in general. When it comes down to it, taking lots of supplements may be marginally better than not taking any at all. But if at all possible, you should get these nutrients and vitamins from actual food and not from a supplement.

You may think that you can find Omega-3 fats in the meat aisle at your local grocery store, which sadly may not be the case. This is because a lot of the meat at grocery stores tends to be sourced from factory farms. Animals that are raised in these farms are not grass-fed in a normal environment, and they are altered with artificial chemicals. Since they are not feeding on natural food like grass, you are not getting these nutrients indirectly as you should. Instead, you are getting artificial chemicals that these animals are fed to make them bigger and thus more profitable for the farm.

They may be expensive, but health grocery stores should be an option that you strongly consider if you want to take autophagy and your body's health seriously. These are places where you can buy meat that does not come from factory farms, and that will have the Omega-3 fats that they should because of it.

Next, we get to the matter of vegetables. Vegetables seem to be the exercise of the food pyramid: everyone knows that it is good, but many people don't like to eat it. If this describes you, you might want to think about using a blender and blending vegetables with fruit so you will eat them.

There are vitamins and nutrients in vegetables that you won't get anywhere else, so it is worthwhile to get yourself to eat them any way that you can. However, be warned that you shouldn't add a lot of fruit, because fruit is high in sugar, which raises your glucose, which prevents autophagy from happening to a significant degree.

You should also think about drinking more green tea. Green tea does a lot of good in making your AMPK go up. While mTOR is the gene that stops autophagy in its tracks, AMPK is the opposite: when stimulated, AMPK will tell your autophagy to turn on.

Green tea makes AMPK go up (and therefore helps to turn on autophagy) particularly well when you couple it with turmeric. Turmeric is actually even more effective in stimulating AMPK, but when you use it together with AMPK, the benefit can only be stronger.

Of all the consumables that I list here, green tea is the most accessible one that will actually make a difference in your autophagy. Green tea helps autophagy because of its active ingredient, EGCG. It is particularly helpful in making autophagy turn on for the liver. Since your liver's health is so important for the general health of your body, drinking green tea every day could make a real difference in living heather and longer.

We also have ginger. Ginger's active ingredient is called 6-shogaol, a chemical that keeps cells in your lungs from being produced too much. This may not be intuitive, but this is actually good for your lungs because it can keep cancer cells from growing too quickly in your lungs, staving off lung cancer. In the meantime, the autophagy you are turning on can clear the chemicals in your lungs that led to cancer cells in the first place.

If you aren't consuming caffeine already, you should really consider it. In specific, caffeine is known to lower your risk for neurodegeneration, which is one of the biggest perks of turning on autophagy. Since you are already getting the process started with autophagy, you might as well maximize your benefits by consuming caffeine.

You won't get autophagy to happen to a satisfactory level with green tea and turmeric alone, but it will help. That goes for all the food items in this chapter. They are not meant to replace all the other big lifestyle changes that will really bring about autophagy. They just help out a lot in making autophagy be the best it can be.

You are not likely to have missed the buzz about CBD oil. If you did, I could fill you in now. CBD is one of the two cannabinoids from the cannabis plant, sometimes referred to as marijuana. However, unlike the other cannabinoid, THC, CBD does not make you high at all. In fact, it does quite the opposite.

Since the cannabis plant was controversial for so long, the research on THC's sister CBD is admittedly limited. However, we do know that CBD leads to less inflammation in the body. CBD even boosts the connections in your brain related to autophagy.

These foods are also great because they are beneficial to your health even outside of autophagy, green tea, and turmeric included.

Our next autophagy-helping food is the reishi mushroom. In the lab, the reishi mushroom was shown to suppress colon cancer cells. This is an interesting case because while there are actually studies showing that autophagy can make cancer cells grow more (cancer cells go through autophagy more), the reishi mushroom has a chemical that stimulates the autophagy of cells that fight against these cancer cells. In most cases, the cancer cells will stop the non-cancer cells from growing, but the reishi mushroom makes sure this doesn't occur.

Coupling fasting with a proper diet in your non-fasting window allows you to cover all your bases with autophagy. Your green tea can increase the potential of autophagy, while turmeric makes it easier to turn on; the reishi mushroom prevents cancer cells from stopping the autophagy of non-cancer cells. These are all things that wouldn't be possible without a proper diet of autophagy-helping foods.

Here are some other foods that you should think about adding to your eating habits: peppers, mushrooms, vinegar, berries, and broccoli. All of these will help you in getting the most possible out of autophagy.

You don't want to only think about autophagy when you pick your foods to eat, though. You still have to think about what is good for your body, after all. Of course, this is not an easy task to do. Plenty of people seem to think they know exactly what you are supposed to eat, despite the fact that everyone knows how much debate there is about what we should eat.

That said, there are some things that we know for sure your body needs, and those are the things we should focus on. A lot of the obvious part is what you should not be eating. Everyone knows not to eat a diet filled with pancakes, Pop-tarts, and chocolate. This is because these foods are filled with calories, which negatively affect your health when consumed in large quantities.

We know of some foods that are always good to choose, like vegetables, unsaturated fats, and a small amount of fruit.

I have told you before that you need to reduce the amount of carbohydrates you have in your diet, but you should also watch the amount of calories you have in general. This will ensure that you will be going in the right direction for your health and body.

Nonetheless, I don't want to lead you to believe that calories are bad, as some do. There is nothing bad about calories in general. In fact, you need calories. It is just that a lot of people forget that it is the nutrients that come from your food that are the most important.

For most people living in the developed world, it is a good idea to try to eat fewer calories, though. Your body has to break down all of the food you eat. Everything that you consume has an effect on your body and your mind. You will fast for less and less time the more calories you eat since you are not able to go through autophagy while your body is digesting. Think about that next time you are about to eat a lot of calories at once.

While you shouldn't only be thinking about foods that turn on autophagy when you decide what to eat, you don't want to eat a lot of foods that slow down autophagy, either. As you know, carbs are your enemy when it comes to getting autophagy going. Your friends are foods that are rich in nutrients.

You also have to make sure your diet has many different kinds of foods. Whether you are fasting to turn on autophagy or not, you can't be healthy without eating all sorts of different foods.

On that note, take the example of craving dessert after eating. Have you ever wondered why there always seems to be room for dessert? The answer to that question is actually three very scientific-sounding words: sensory-specific satiety.

Scientists have been studying people's eating habits in a quest to understand the answer to this conundrum. It turns out that our body has a mechanism to get us a eat many different types of foods. This is meant to prevent us from eating a lot of one food without getting other nutrients from different sources.

Your body tells you to eat ice cream after you say you are full-on one food because of sensory-selective satiety. Hunger can feel like an objective measure of how much you can be eating, but this phenomenon shows us that it is not as black and white as all that. Hunger tells us to eat different kinds of food when we eat too much of one thing. Unfortunately, we have not yet evolved to crave only healthy foods and to avoid unhealthy ones, but this is still a useful mechanism to get us to do what is good for us by not eating only one food.

It is also vital that you make sure to get plenty of Vitamin D from whatever source you can. Vitamin D is essential to a lot of things that our bodies do, and autophagy is one of them. You may not even realize how important Vitamin D is. If you don't get sufficient Vitamin D, there are very real and significant consequences for your autophagy. As a result, the autophagy that you go through will not detox your cells nearly as well as they should.

The good thing is that it is easy to get plenty of this important Vitamin by getting plenty of sun. The sun will provide all of this vitamin that you will need, so if you live somewhere where it is sunny most of the time, this won't be a problem for you. As long as you are sure to use sunscreen to protect your epidermis from harmful ultraviolet rays, you will be safe and get the exposure of Vitamin D that your autophagy requires. If you don't live somewhere sunny, there are still other ways to get Vitamin D.

You can get Vitamin D from a lot of different foods, including milk, or you can even take a supplement for it. However, as you know, we always recommend that you get your vitamins from a food source rather than from a supplement.

One of the reasons that all of the foods we listed are good for your autophagy is that they lower your energy levels. This may not sound like a good thing at first. After all, one of the main perks of turning on autophagy is supposed to be having higher energy levels.

In this context, I am referring to lowering the energy levels of your cells, which is something that all of your cells do. When this happens, your cells have a great chance of entering a state of stress, and you know what that leads to.

As a result, your cells will start breaking down their damaged organelles, proteins, and foreign toxins. Not only that, but every food mentioned in this chapter is particularly healthy for your neurons. Everyone wants to make sure to keep up the health of their brain, so this is a great benefit to have.

We have not yet gotten to the importance of healthy, unsaturated fats in a diet of someone who wants to turn on autophagy. People who start going into ketosis from the keto diet go through a great amount of autophagy when they are sleeping, and it is all because their systems are filled with these healthy fats.

Why exactly are healthy fats such an important part of your new diet? It is because unsaturated fats do the important work of absorbing nutrients like vitamins and minerals. Fats also help in constructing membranes and membranes that protect your nerves from damage. In addition to that, your fats help you move your muscles, keep your blood from clotting, and prevent inflammation in your body.

I have mentioned that unsaturated fats are healthy, and saturated fats are not, but it's time that you learned how exactly that works. Not all fats are created equally. The healthy fats that you want to get plenty of are called polyunsaturated and monounsaturated fats. These fats are always good (unless, of course, you go to extremes, which is always the case with nutrition).

Next, we have trans fats. Trans fats are now banned in many countries, including the United States. The reason they are so harmful is that they provide no health benefit whatsoever while leading to clogging in the blood and an increased risk of inflammation. Trans fat does not occur in nature, either; it is actually the byproduct of artificial processes used to package and preserve food. Clearly, you don't want any trans-fat in your diet.

Finally, our last fat is the saturated fats. If we had to say they were good or bad, we would say that saturated fats are basically bad. However, it is not as if it is poisonous, so it is OK to have a little bit of saturated fat. You just don't want to eat more than a small amount of it, and you probably don't even want to eat it every day.

The worst types of fats are trans fats and saturated fats, while polyunsaturated and monounsaturated fats are the healthy ones that you should eat.

Nutritionists say that around one-third of your calories should come out of good fats like polyunsaturated and monounsaturated fats. You can see what kinds of fats you are eating by looking at the labels on the foods you eat. Since the goods fats are what you are aiming for, make sure you buy plenty of foods like fatty fish, nuts, seeds, and even veggies. These healthy fats are also found in flaxseed.

Since fish is not a common dish in all settings, it can be surprising for some people that the American Heart Association says we should be eating two meals with fatty fish every single week. Healthy fats are so good for us that we should be going out of our way to get them.

Sadly, trans fats and carbohydrates are a normal part of the American diet. Trans fats may not be legal anymore, but we still see plenty of artificial chemicals on the labels of popular snack foods, and these chemicals are probably no better. It should go without saying that you need to avoid packaged snack foods like the plague. They will hinder your autophagy tremendously. We see these chemicals in pastries, fried goods, sugary icing, saltines, brownies, false butter, and more.

What makes healthy fats so important, though? Your blood starts to cause congestion in our veins and arteries, especially as we age. The role of unsaturated fats is helping to unclog them. If you don't get enough healthy fat in your diet, particularly as we get older, you are looking at higher risks for conditions that are caused by clogged arteries.

When it comes to saturated fats, even though they are not completely bad like trans fats, we still don't want to be eating these fats as much as most of us do. You would be surprised by how much-saturated fats get into your diet without you even thinking about it. Doctors tell us that at most, we should be getting 10% of our calories from saturated fats on a daily basis. If you can, you should aim to eat even less saturated fat.

Trans fats and saturated fats both, to different extents, make your cholesterol go up, make your heart disease risk go up, and clog your veins and arteries. As usual, it is worth mentioning that these risks also go up the older you get. That's why it is essential to pay attention to the kinds of fats you are eating every day.

The diet in Mediterranean culture is famous for being high in unsaturated fat, from olive oil in specific. People living in this area are also famous for having a record-breaking low level of heart disease. They are what led nutritionists to learn more about unsaturated fats, eventually, determine that not all fats are bad. Some are actually vital.

Polyunsaturated fats are common in vegetable oil. Vegetable oil is well known for making your cholesterol go down. Omega-3 fats are also considered a polyunsaturated fat. The thing that makes lowering your saturated fat intake easier is that you can often replace the foods with high saturated fat with foods with high unsaturated fat. Any time you have the option to do this, do it. Your heart and arteries will thank you.

If you are going to start consuming more olive oil for the polyunsaturated fats, you do have to be careful, because not every bottle of olive oil is created equal. There is an unfortunate number of olive oil companies that do not use real, natural ingredients for it, meaning you will not get the health benefits from it that you should.

Polyunsaturated fats are a special case for fats because your body is not able to produce these kinds of fats without consuming them. That, and your body actually needs them for various biological processes.

Meanwhile, saturated and trans fats are terrible for your cholesterol. In higher than low amounts, saturated fats lead to blocked arteries, which puts you at risk for health problems.

Despite the common misconception, the amount of fat that you consume does not affect your risk for diseases like cancer. What does affect your risk of cancer is overweight or obese, and this is more likely to happen if you are consuming too many trans and saturated fats, or if you are consuming too much fat overall.

It would be a disservice to talk about diet in the context of autophagy without talking about the health risks associated with being obese or overweight. If you belong to the demographic of overweight women who have already gone through menopause, you should be aware of this risk, especially. People in this demographic can significantly lower their risks for diseases related to weight by following our advice.

The way that you feel subjectively will start to change as a result of fasting and following this new diet. The reason is that hunger has a strong relationship with blood sugar levels. The more glucose you have in your blood, the less you crave food because your system feels like it has enough of it.

Chapter 7
Metabolic Autophagy in Practice

Now armed with tons of knowledge about autophagy and how to take advantage of its effects on your body, you might still be unsure where to begin. It is understandable; after all, it is a lot of information to take in. That's why this chapter is about starting up metabolic autophagy in practice and how to avoid making the same mistakes many autophagy practitioners make when trying to turn on autophagy. To begin, you should consider how many people start living their lives aware of autophagy but give up on harnessing its potential very fast. The key to using autophagy to its highest potential is to start slow and be consistent.

To begin, you should consider how many people start living their lives aware of autophagy but give up on harnessing its potential very fast. The key to using autophagy to its highest potential is to start slow and be consistent.

But we have already discussed the importance of having the right mindset when learning about water fasting. Still, there is one component of turning on autophagy that you cannot underestimate, or you will regret it. And that is sleep.

Sleep is so important to autophagy that it is the first topic in the chapter about turning on autophagy in practice. Even outside the context of autophagy, sleep is a mysterious thing. Not even scientists or psychologists know what it is for. They have guessed that it is for the brain rather than the body, but other than that, they do not know why we even do it.

While sleeping alone doesn't turn on autophagy, you truly shouldn't underestimate the importance of sleep in getting the most out of it. We want to turn on autophagy for our overall health, too, and sleep is an incredibly important part of our overall health.

If you are not getting eight hours of sleep every night, you are not ready to turn on autophagy whenever you can. That's because missing out on sleep is so bad for you that you might as well not do something healthy like fasting to turn on autophagy.

Sleeping is the most important time of the day for autophagy. This is when your body is fixing all the damage you have accumulated, after all, and since autophagy is necessary any time you are repairing, sleep is a crucial time for it. Another reason that sleep is so important for autophagy is that your body isn't using energy for much else at this point. This makes it a good time for processes like autophagy to take place. You aren't using energy to digest, move, talk, or do anything, so your body can take advantage of that and get as much out of the time as possible.

That means if you aren't getting the recommended eight hours of sleep every night, you are egregiously lowering the amount of work that autophagy could be doing on your body.

And this is not even talking about serious sleep deprivation. If you sleep for only six hours instead of eight, sometimes, this is something you should work on improving, too. But some people get even less sleep than that, and this is a problem. The less sleep you get, the less autophagy you are getting in your body. If you have a habit of doing this over time, this creates problems for your health and immune system.

This is not even to mention all of the negative side effects of sleep deprivation that are unrelated to autophagy. Being short on sleep leads to cravings, a lack of clarity of thought, low executive functioning control, and a less efficient metabolism.

To keep things elegant, you should try to think of your time sleeping every night as doing the opposite work of eating during the day. If you spend 4 hours during the day eating, your body spends 8 hours a day breaking all of that down at night.

Depending on the nutritional value of the food, your number of hours breaking down food in autophagy every night could be different, but the point is that your body has to take care of all the chemicals you put in it. This is what your eight hours of sleep are for, and if you aren't getting them, you are hindering the proper functions of your system in a major way.

The complementary period of time to your sleep is what happens when you get up in the morning. While you should be breaking down your food from the previous day in autophagy while you sleep, the next morning, you should eat more than you eat for the rest of the day.

This is not a common thing to do in all cultures, but it is actually the smartest thing to do because your body is better at breaking food down in the morning and earlier in the day.

If you want to go above and beyond, you should really try to go to bed earlier on days that you do a serious fast. If you go to bed early and on an empty stomach, you will be optimizing the autophagy in your cells.

I recommend going to bed earlier because this will help you have more deep sleep or REM sleep. Most of the autophagy that occurs while you are asleep happens during this phase of sleep, so you should try to get as much deep sleep as possible.

Finally, try to maximize the amount of melatonin in your brain when you sleep. Melatonin is essential for turning on autophagy in your brain cells, giving you yet another reason to prioritize sleep if you care about autophagy.

That means it makes the most sense to fit in as many nutrients as you can in the morning, so your stomach can break them down efficiently.

It can be hard to get a good night's sleep these days for a variety of reasons. Back when we lived in caves, we didn't have these problems because the sun went down and we all simply had no choice but to go to bed and wait for the light to come back.

Since we have so many things to do and so many bright lights competing for our attention, getting to bed at a reasonable hour has become an increasingly more difficult task.

Studies show that the blue lights emanating from our screens are detrimental to our sleep. If you care about the quality of your sleep, and if you care about getting to sleep at a reasonable time, you need to find a way to manage the blue lights around you at night. Ideally, you don't interact with your smartphone or laptop at all before you hit the hay.

The next time the sun goes down, I challenge you to accept that to mean it is night time, meaning you don't look at any screens after that happens. You will find that this is almost impossible to do these days. It doesn't help that a lot of us have our work on these gadgets too.

Since it is so hard to deal with blue lights the ideal way, you may have to compromise so you can still sleep as well as you can for your autophagy. If you wear glasses, you can wear special lenses that block out some of the blue light from devices. You can also adjust brightness settings, making your screens darker or sometimes even turning off blue light entirely.

The important thing to know is that if you don't look at these screens before bed, you will see a big difference in the quality of your sleep.

What to Avoid in Your First Fast

Since you are reading a book about fasting before you do it, you get the privilege of learning from other people's mistakes before making these mistakes on your own. Don't make the same mistakes other people make, because you can learn from them now and avoid them later.

Of course, you are bound to make some of the same mistakes. We are all just human. However, equipped with the experiences of others, you can do your best not to repeat the same mistakes.

One big mistake that almost everyone makes does not have long enough fasts. Don't forget that fact we talked about earlier in the book: if you eat a low-carb meal before your fast, you are still digesting it for four hours afterward; if you have a meal with a good amount of carbs before fasting, it takes 8 hours to digest. While you are digesting, you are not in autophagy.

It seems that very few autophagy practitioners are aware of this very helpful fact. They believe they are fasting for 12 hours, but they are really fasting for 8. If they are really out of the loop and not avoiding carbs, that 12-hour fast turns into a 4-hour fast. This little principle can really change the way you think about your fasts.

Of course, there is still value to these shorter fasts, given that you are not eating 4 hours before bed. If you get full autophagy during a full night of sleep, in addition to getting autophagy during the day, you are still doing good by your body. It doesn't matter if it only calculates to be a 4-hour fast after digestion — even that will have a positive effect on your health.

But this is where the value of the water fast really shines because once you become aware of this harsh mathematical reality, you might wish to get more out of your fasting.

All things considered, I would say that short fasts may not be a common mistake, but rather a common opportunity for improvement. You could settle for the daily 4-hour fast with intermittent fasting, but you could also go for more and try to do a 24-hour water fast every other week. You know everything you need to know to do it after reading — what's stopping you from trying?

There are writers on this subject who say that there is no reason to fast for more than 12 hours. However, scientific studies on the matter don't support this idea. In fact, research shows that those who go for 24 hours fasting had 300% more autophagosomes in their bodies. When they went for 12 hours longer, autophagosomes went up 20% more.

As you can see, the number of autophagosomes (and therefore, the level of autophagy) increases astronomically 24 hours into a fast. This level of autophagosomes reaches its highest point at 36 hours, but it doesn't increase nearly as much as it did before.

Again, though, that doesn't mean there is no reason to fast for longer than 24 or 36 hours. Your cells are breaking down toxins and rebuilding cell structures the entire time that you are doing autophagy, so you are still getting this benefit. And as you stay in this level of autophagy for longer, you really notice a difference in how you feel, compared to just going through autophagy when you sleep.

Your takeaway here should be that the biggest increase in autophagy happens after 24 hours of fasting, while the highest level of autophagy happens at 36 hours. You should memorize this fact and take your own health status and goals into consideration to decide the way you want to fast.

As we said before, you will definitely see improvements in your health even if you only do a daily 12-hour fast. I am only telling you about how much more autophagy you get from 24 hours so you can get some perspective, and perhaps to convince you to challenge yourself with a water fast, if your body can safely handle it.

Although your autophagosomes do not increase as nearly as much after 24 hours, you will still continue to be at a very high caliber of autophagy that will do your body a lot of good. Your cells will continue to be detoxified the whole time.

So the first big mistake people make is doing fasts that are too short. The next big mistake is not doing fasts frequently enough. People who make this mistake seem to think that doing a few very intense fasts every year is going to make their bodies healthy, but they are wrong. Once again, I have to repeat that consistency is everything when we are talking about autophagy.

Consistency isn't just about turning on autophagy every day, either. It also means being consistent in your health, and not just expecting one healthy thing that you do to turn on autophagy is going to be enough to make you a healthy individual. Sleep was our example earlier: what is the point of someone who fasts for autophagy if they are running off of six hours of sleep every night? That person still isn't healthy.

You may have an idea of the next aspect of health I am going to bring up in regard to consistency: exercise. It truly seems like exercise is the very last thing that anyone wants to do, but it is extremely good for you to get regular exercise. There is even some solid evidence to suggest that exercise rivals fasting in terms of turning on autophagy the most effectively.

We have an entire chapter devoted to exercising and autophagy, but it is still good to think about it in terms of how it fits together with fasting. No matter if you are overweight, skinny, or athletic, you have to find time to work out on days that you fast. Even if you only work out for fifteen minutes, that's fifteen minutes more of exercise that you didn't have before. That's how valuable exercise is to your health.

Studies on mice have proved the viability of exercise to turn on autophagy. When mice were running in the lab, and scientists measured their level of autophagosomes afterward, they were found to have high levels of autophagosomes after the exercise. Exercises like cardio, therefore, are known to be a good way to turn on autophagy.

Without digging too much into the exercise chapter, there is actually evidence that strength/resistance training is more effective in turning on autophagy than cardio. You can work on your muscles to reduce tissue loss while also turning on autophagy.

It is strange that cardio is always so emphasized since there is a lot of evidence that strength/resistance training could be even better for you. Of course, cardio is great for your body too, but maybe the real reason that cardio gets such a focus is that it is seen as the best way to lose weight.

So far, I have told you to avoid fasting not long enough, avoid not fasting consistently, and to avoid not exercising. You could sum that up as fast for long enough, fast often enough, and don't forget to exercise.

There is another common mistake with fasting that connects to our discussion about the mental aspect of water fasting, as well as to the issue of fasting with consistency. To put it in few words, in order to succeed with intermittent fasting — or any fast, really — you have to resist the temptation to give up.

We said it before: it is easy to start things, but following through with them is another story.

I won't repeat the part about needing to keep a clear goal, but that still applies here. To avoid giving up before you can even start, you need to start out with small goals. You could even call them easy goals. The easiest starting point for intermittent fasting and keeping yourself from eating after dinner at 6pm.

If you do that, a 12-hour fast only requires you to wait until 6am the next morning to eat. (As you know, this is really an 8-hour fast, but for the sake of ease, we will keep calling them their normal lengths without considering digestion.)

Once you have a hang of the shorter fast, you can go for the longer ones.

The key to success and safety with the water fast is going into it with your goals clearly defined. Ask yourself right now, since you are pretty far into the book at this point: what are you doing this for? Do you want to lose weight? Do you want to look younger? Do you want to live longer?

While it's true that autophagy achieves all three for you, you still need to have a purpose for autophagy that is for you and you alone. If you don't, you won't be very likely to change entire aspects of your lifestyle for it. Once you have a well-defined purpose for something, all the rest starts to fall into place, because you know what you want to do.

The opposite of that is when you don't have a well-defined purpose at all, and you give up easily. If you don't know why you're doing something, it is very easy for you to give up on it. You don't even have a point in continuing with it, so why wouldn't you?

It is very easy to start things. Anyone can start a 300-word novel. Anyone can start a sculpture. What makes you accomplished is when you can start something and finish it. Autophagy and water fasting is no different. If you have a clear reason you want to see through your first water fast to the end, you will be far less likely to fall out of it.

Having your goal in mind isn't just a preventive measure against giving up; it's almost a way for you to do things the right way. If you are in the middle of a water fast, you might be tempted to get a snack, even though you know it ruins the purpose of the entire fast. When you already know your goal for water fasting, though, you are a lot less likely to fall for temptations like these.

You can tell yourself, "I am fasting to lose weight. I won't lose weight if I add more food into my stomach during this fast, so I'm not going to cheat on the fast with that cookie."

Alternatively, if you went into your water fast without a goal like this, things would probably go a lot different. You would see the cookie and say, "Well, it is my first day fasting. I can do things the correct way next time." Since you don't have a clear reason for water fasting, there just isn't that emotional weight to cheating on the fast that there otherwise would be.

A second crucial but often overlooked part of the mindset of someone who succeeds in the water fast is knowledge of fasts and autophagy. Plenty of people believe they know things about these topics, so much that they actually do fasting the way they believe is correct, whether it is right or not.

Fortunately, you have this whole book of easy-to-understand information about fasting and autophagy. You could return to it if you need to know more, but chances are, you are absorbing it so well that it isn't even necessary. You already have this second crucial part of the mindset covered.

Finally, there is the third and last part of the mindset required to succeed in a water fast, and it is adaptability. You have lots of goals that propelled you to do a water fast in the first place, but the one that will carry the fate of all the others is your adaptability to a new, healthier way of living. This mental aspect will determine if you continue water fasting a few times a month, or if it is just something you do one time and never again.

You will get some health benefits from the autophagy that comes from water fasting one time, but these benefits are pointless if you don't keep it up. That's why it's so crucial that you adapt well to the new habits you formed and do it again in a few weeks.

Chapter 8
Autophagy and Training
to Build Muscle

There is some research to back the claim that resistance training — that is, muscle-building exercises — turn on autophagy in your body even more than fasting. When you are at the gym using your muscles, you are making tiny tears in your muscle tissue that your cells have to repair using the process of autophagy.

A lot of people are hesitant to go to the gym at all, let alone do more intense exercise like resistance training. But if you want to get as much out of your body's autophagy as possible, your efforts are best spent in working out your muscles.

After seven chapters about the food you put into your body, we can finally focus on something that is equally important to autophagy: exercise. We have brought it up again and again, but we have not yet gone in-depth on what makes it such a vital part of turning on autophagy.

Exercise is such an effective method of turning on autophagy that it is perfectly valid to choose it as your main method of doing so. However, most people will not choose to do this because exercising regularly is much harder to keep up than intermittent fasting.

As always, the best option is doing a combination of both: fasting and exercising. If you do your daily 8 hour fast before your run on the treadmill, you will increase your autophagy much more than if you did just one or the other.

If you still aren't sure if exercise isn't important for autophagy, consider the study showing that those who did strength exercises for twenty minutes had higher levels of autophagosomes than those who fasted for 36 hours.

It can be hard to believe, but this is what bearer out in science. This is so hard to accept, since it may be true that mostly no one wants to exercise. How could it be true that exercise is more effective in turning on autophagy than fasting?

It may be a comfort to know that, in a way, fasting is still more effective than normally turning on autophagy through exercising. That's because exercise is a challenging thing to keep doing on a routine basis.

A lot of people get excited about fasting, only to quit eventually. You can imagine how much worse this phenomenon is with working out. If exercise was the way that most people turned on autophagy, hardly anyone would be getting the benefits of it.

Thankfully, we have intermittent fasting available to us as our main path to autophagy. However, since this is a book about doing what is best for our health and our bodies, we still need to at least learn about what exercise can do for our natural detox agent.

Remember that autophagy is not really ever "on" or "off." There is always some autophagy going on in your body, in some organ or another. Talking about "turning on autophagy" is just a simpler way of saying that we want to make your autophagy reach more significant goals for our bodies than it would if we didn't intentionally "turn it on."

This means we are not literally trying to turn on autophagy — it is always on to some degree. It is that degree that we are trying to influence: we want to turn on autophagy to the highest degree possible using fasting, the keto diet, and exercise.

The "regular" level of autophagy is often called the maintenance mode by experts. The maintenance mode is the amount of autophagy that everyone gets, even if they have no clue what autophagy even means.

When we say, "turn on autophagy," we really mean "turn on advanced autophagy." We mean go from maintenance mode autophagy to advanced autophagy.

Fasting alone will certainly get you to the level of advanced autophagy, but you can go even further than that. You will want to once you become enamored by the energy autophagy gives you the weight it helps you lose and the quality of skin that it restores for you.

You shouldn't think that either fasting or exercise is pointless just because one alone will do the trick. Truthfully, you are probably best off picking one or the other in the beginning, so you don't get burnt out. Of course, intermittent fasting is always your best choice to avoid this consequence. But you will have this chapter as a resource to go back to once you start to see the positive effects autophagy has on your body and you want to have even more of it.

The Health of the Individual who Exercises to Increase Autophagy

The average person who exercises regularly probably does not know about autophagy, just like the average person, in general, doesn't know about autophagy. But it's not only the benefits of exercise overall that makes it good for you. Autophagy specifically will see positive consequences as a result of your regular exercise.

For one, in people who exercise, autophagosomes are at much higher counts than people who do not exercise. Scientists saw this in an experiment that paid attention to the autophagy levels of athletes and non-athletes. To no one's surprise, the athletes had more autophagosomes than the control group.

You should be able to look at this from the other side, though. There are benefits to the autophagy that fasting offers that exercise does not. For one, in mice that fasted to turn on autophagy, skeletal muscle fibers were strengthened. The mice could stop their muscle fibers from degrading because autophagy from fasting could stop dysfunctional organelles from building up. Mice who turned on autophagy through exercise did not see this benefit at all.

The point is that fasting and exercise both turn on autophagy, but they don't always turn on the same kind of autophagy. You can't go wrong by turning on autophagy through both means.

Another example has to do with the equilibrium of your muscles when you exercise. It can be hard for your body to keep them at equilibrium, but if you fast, the autophagy that is triggered can greatly help in maintaining equilibrium.

If you fast as well as exercise, you will also see a greater count of collagen in your skin cells, the protein they produce that keeps your skin elastic. If you do only one or the other, you do not see as great of an effect.

It goes to show you that while exercise may be shown to turn on higher levels of autophagy in a shorter amount of time, the autophagy that you are looking for is not always achieved through either means. You don't have to decide on just one; when the time comes that you realize the benefits autophagy gives you, decide to do both.

Maybe the best benefit that combining the two can give you is in dealing with loose skin that can come from weight loss. In a study where people who lost weight with either fasting, exercising, or both, the respondents who said they did both had less loose skin than those who turned on autophagy with just one method or the other.

This loose skin is often referred to as a "skin curtain," and many people will even say that they are hesitant to lose weight because of the threat of loose skin.

There is a lot of misinformation out there about loose skin, so it is understandable that people would be concerned about it. But loose skin doesn't have to be a sure thing; it all depends on how quickly you lose weight, your level of hydration, your level of autophagy, and your age.

Three out of four of these things are completely in your control. If you make sure to drink plenty of water, pace yourself in your exercise routine and fasting, and use all the methods we describe in this book to maximize your autophagy, your loose skin fears won't be as horrible as you might imagine.

The "skin curtain" is often seen in people who lose weight without considering autophagy as part of the equation. You see, autophagy helps against the threat of loose skin because autophagy is all about your cells eating dead cells to use them for raw materials and replace them with new cells. If you are keeping up a healthy level of autophagy while you are losing weight, by the time you lose the weight and your skin has to readjust, it will be able to do so much more easily. All because your cells were taken care of through autophagy. Autophagy keeps your skin tight and youthful, no matter how much weight you lose.

It is surprising that we have not even talked much about skin, yet to this point, but the chapter on exercise is an excellent opportunity to do it. Your skin will truly give off a new glow if you make autophagy a new part of your routine, but this is doubly true if you make exercise a part of your autophagy routine.

At the end of the day, though, skin is usually a matter of cosmetics, much like weight can be. If you are more concerned about your health and risk for age-related disease, exercise is still a good choice for autophagy stimulation. This is because exercise is the best way you can lower the inflammation in your body, pretty close to diet and fasting.

Your inflammation may be pretty high, depending on the healthiness of your previous lifestyle. People who ate poorly before, smoked, were mostly sedentary, or drank a lot are at higher risk of high inflammation. Fortunately, exercise is so powerful that it can reverse inflammation that results from all of these factors. Inflammation is the source of a lot of risks for age-related disease, so reducing it is always a good idea.

Your body overall performs better when you don't have as much inflammation. Chronic inflammation, in particular, is what will make you start to see the beginning symptoms of different age-related diseases.

Exercise doesn't have to be as painful as you might envision it to be in your mind. Just like with fasting, you have to start small and work your way up to more ambitious goals.

Keep your goals written down in a notebook that you can look at every day. Do this from the very beginning, so you don't lose sight of what you are trying to do with autophagy and exercise.

Your first task is to follow through with the first action step of your fitness plan. If you can follow through with it for a few weeks, this is when you start to work towards higher goals.

We said that you might go from an 8-hour fast to a 10-hour fast. With exercise, the situation is almost the same. You might start out telling yourself to go to the gym once a week for thirty minutes (or less, depending on your level of fitness). After you are able to follow through with this small goal for a few weeks, write down that you want to go to the gym for thirty minutes twice a week. Once you can follow through with the second goal consistently for a few weeks, build on that one. You get the idea; you have to start small with your goals if you expect to actually achieve them.

Finally, you have to think about what kind of exercise you are going to do. There are experts who tell you there are a dozen different kinds of ways to work out, but to keep things simple, we can really say there are just three: cardio, core, and resistance.

Cardio is running, biking, endurance, and so on. These are exercises that test the capacity of your lungs and how long you can strain yourself physically. There have been tests on mice that show they went through significant autophagy because of cardio, so this is a valid way to go.

Core exercises are less tested in the context of autophagy, but we know that physical activity, in general, is good for autophagy, so we can basically assume it turns on autophagy as well.

Finally, we have resistance training. Some people call this strength training. Resistance training is all about using your muscles, lifting weights, and increasing your strength. There is actually valid new research suggesting that resistance training is the best method of turning on autophagy out of all of them.

Cardio was demonstrated to make the number of autophagosomes in mice go up, but resistance training was demonstrated to make autophagy turn on even more. This means that working on your muscles is probably the best way to turn on autophagy.

Of course, we still have to consider practicality. Practicality is what makes intermittent fasting still take the cake when it comes to the best way to turn on autophagy, just because far more people are going to be willing to abstain from eating for hours a day than are work on their arms every other day.

Resistance training is so good for autophagy because it puts your cells through long periods of stress, especially in your muscles cells. When your cells are in this state, they go into their resources of cellular garbage to get energy. If you do resistance training exercises over time, your cells are going through high levels of autophagy for a long period of time, and it really gets your autophagosomes to come out.

Not only that, but this kind of autophagy will keep you from seeing as much muscle loss as you get older. When you have more muscle mass, this is an indication that you have better general health; when you are in better shape already, your autophagy is better too. This is why resistance training is so effective in turning on this natural detoxifier.

You may be familiar with the relaxed feeling you get after you do strength exercises. Part of this feeling is the rush of endorphins you get in your brain, as these are your body's natural pain relievers. But the other reason for this feeling is from the tiny tears that you make in your muscles when you use them.

The kind of stress that resistance training puts you in is the perfect kind for turning on autophagy: short-term acute stress. The most straightforward way to achieve it is by simply lifting weights. If you think you can take it, you would be doing yourself a great service by doing weight lifting every day for about 30 minutes. That may seem like a lot, but the benefits your body would reap from it would far outweigh the negatives you feel from doing it.

A Note before the Conclusion

There are many things that make the autophagy-centered lifestyle different from other health practices. One of them is the simplicity of doing it. When you follow the keto diet, the only things you need to pay attention to on the nutritional label are carbohydrates and the kinds of fats. Compared to other diets, this requires very little of you.

Fasting is even simpler. You don't have to count calories, because you have to stay away from them completely. I'm not saying this is easy, but the hard rule of "don't eat for 24 hours" is very straightforward.

Fasting can be hard for people at first, but you will probably be surprised. People tend to find it to be easier than they expected.

If you fail at your first fast, consider shortening your goal, from 16 hours to 12 hours, for example. There is no rush in developing your fasting routine. When you induce autophagy, you are going the extra mile for your body. Be proud of yourself for that and let yourself take it slow.

Sometimes the mind can seem like a mystical thing that is impossible to understand, so let's touch briefly on your brain and how it fits into building these new habits.

Much like autophagy, the study of the brain has made great progress in the past decade. Now we know that the cells in your brain (called neurons) are connected to one another with trillions of connections, called synapses.

This is a tremendous discovery. The discovery of synapses tells us that the connections in our brain change constantly, depending on the inputs we give it. If you create new habits like fasting once a week, eating new foods, and exercising regularly, you are creating new connections in your brain. Once these connections have been solidly established (which takes about a month or so, just like a habit), living your life a new way will just feel normal.

Conclusion

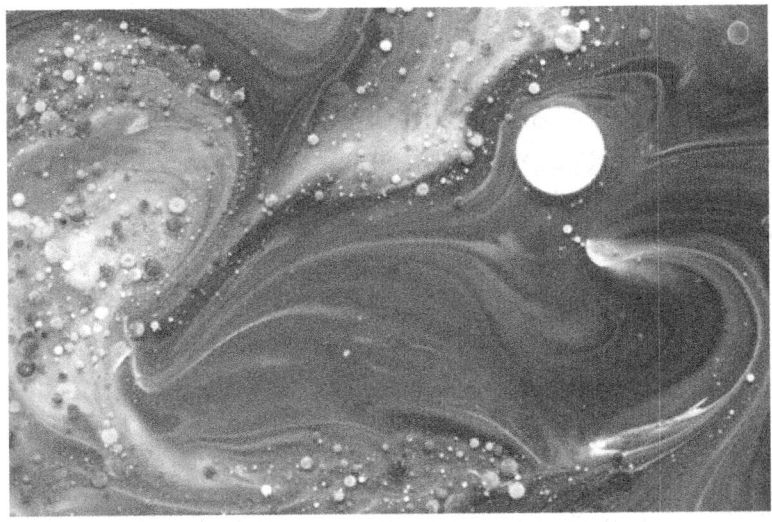

Thank you for making it through to the end of *Autophagy*, let's hope it was informative and able to provide you with all of the tools you need to achieve your goals whatever they may be.

Scientists are not finished making discoveries about the potential healing powers of autophagy, but they have found out enough about this biological process to tell us that turning on autophagy in your body is a great thing to do for your health. The health of your cells is the health of your body, so keeping your cells free of toxins and thus running more smoothly has all sorts of positive health consequences. People who turn on autophagy have lower inflammation, weigh less, have lower blood pressure, and have generally better biomarkers.

For most people, intermittent fasting is the best option for turning on your autophagy. You have read about the variety of techniques that will also have this effect on your body, but intermittent fasting is the most practical one for several reasons. If you made exercise your main path to achieving autophagy, it is more likely than not, you would fall out of your workout routine and lose all the benefits of autophagy. If the keto diet was your main path towards regular autophagy, there is a good chance that you would not keep this up either.

You won't run into this issue with intermittent fasting because it requires nothing but a small adjustment in your day-to-day life: the time that you eat. With all that said, you should absolutely shoot for exercising and dieting in a way to turn on autophagy in addition to intermittent fasting. I am only recommending intermittent fasting as a jumping-off point. Once you are in the routine of fasting, you will probably feel motivated to maximize your body's natural detoxifier in other ways, too.

I hope this book has helped you learn how to aim for higher things for your health and body. If you are curious to learn more about the science of autophagy, look no further than the appendix at the back of the book.

Finally, if you found this book useful in any way, a review on Amazon is always appreciated!

Appendix
Scientific studies on autophagy, intermittent fasting and related subjects

Alirezaei, Kemball, Flynn, Wood, Whitton Kiosses. *Short-term fasting induces profound neuronal autophagy.* Published online 2010 Aug 14.

ncbi.nlm.nih.gov/pmc/articles/PMC3106288/

The researchers in this study watched the autophagosomes — collectors of material to be broken down in autophagy — of cells of people who fasted. They found that the number of autophagosomes increased significantly in people who fasted and that as a result, they had an increase of autophagy in their brains. Autophagy is known to have a profoundly beneficial effect on the brain in the context of neurodegenerative disease.

Finnell, Saul, Goldhamer, Myers. *Is fasting safe? A chart review of adverse effects during medically supervised, water-only fasting.* Published 2018 February 20. ncbi.nlm.nih.gov/pmc/articles/PMC5819235/

The article starts out conceding that water fasting has been proved to have some health benefits. The author felt there was a lack of research on potential negative consequences of water fasting, which is the subject of this experiment. The conclusion after testing patients on water fasting was that it was safe enough to use as treatment in a controlled setting.

Francoise, Grundler, Bergouignan, Dorinda, Michalsen. *Safety, health improvement, and well-being during a 4 to 21-day fasting period in an observational study including 1422 subjects.* Published 2019 Jan 2. ncbi.nlm.nih.gov/pmc/articles/PMC6314618/

This study aims to study subjects who are not obese who do fasting over a long period of time. The main measurements were the health changes of the subject as well as their safety over the span of a year. Even over the course of a year, there were significant and measurable differences in weight, waist size, and blood pressure. The subjects increased improved well-being, both physically and emotionally. They expressed a diminished feeling of hunger as well. Fewer than 1% expressed safety concerns from the experiment, and over 80% said they noticed improvements in health.

Ganesan, Habboush, Sultan. *Intermittent Fasting: The Choice for a Healthy Lifestyle*. Published online 2018 July 9. ncbi.nlm.nih.gov/pmc/articles/PMC6128599/

Says that the basic reduction of food consumption leads to weight loss. Looked at over 800 studies about intermittent fasting done in the last two decades, and takes note of the fact that only 4 of all of these meet the criteria required to be considered entirely scientific, such as having a control group. Still, the study says that an increase in fat loss was a consistent trend in these studies. IF is determined to be an effective way of losing weight, but says that more research is needed to say any more.

Stockman, Thomas, Burke, Apovian. *Intermittent Fasting: Is the Wait Worth the Weigh?* Published online 2019 June 1.

ncbi.nlm.nih.gov/pmc/articles/PMC5959807/

A meta-study of research done about the effects of intermittent fasting on both animals and humans. Note that IF is difficult to study since many variations of it exist. Says that the results can also vary as a result, although there is a consistent conclusion that IF leads to weight loss and improved biomarker. Even showed that in animals, IF led to less of oxidative stress, better cognition, and slowed aging. Said there were anti-inflammatory effects as well.

Templeman, Gonzalez, Thompson, Betts. *The role of intermittent fasting and meal timing in weight management and metabolic health*. Published 2019 April 26. ncbi.nlm.nih.gov/pubmed/31023390

Centered around the problem of obesity as a public health issue, this study seeks to find solutions, postulating that intermittent fasting may be one. Looks into the effectiveness of fasting in general without assuming that it must be good. They concluded that fasting longer than 16 hours, in particular, showed some physiological difference in the people who participated, including fat loss and insulin control. The paper says that the reason for this change could be caloric restriction rather than fasting.

Intermittent Fasting for Women 101

The Ultimate Step-by-Step Guide for Weight Loss, Even If You Are Over 50, with the Keto Diet, 16/8 Method and Self-Cleansing Through the Metabolic Process of Autophagy

Jennifer Cook

Introduction

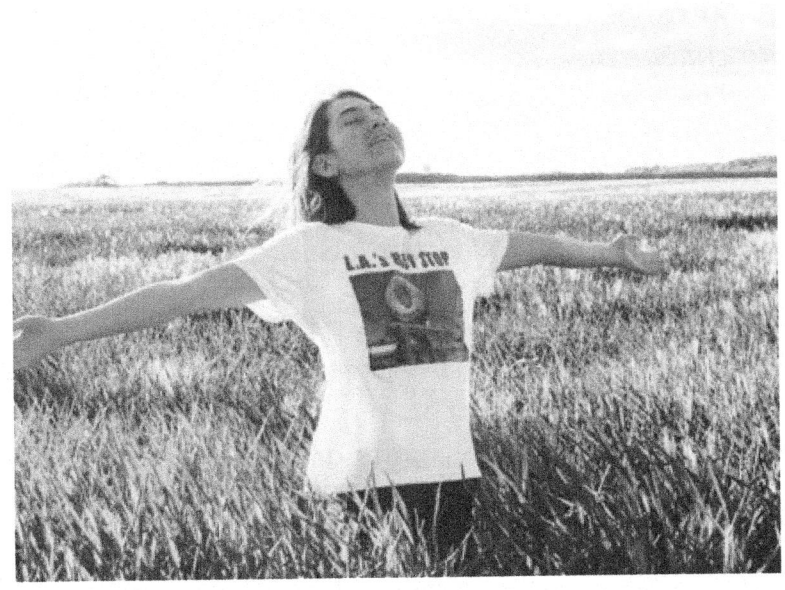

Congratulations on purchasing *Intermittent Fasting for Women 101* and thank you for doing so.

Intermittent fasting is a method of eating that any woman can use to lose weight and achieve a healthier body. Unlike in traditional fasting, intermittent fasting allows you to cycle between periods of eating and not eating. Doing so activates a biological process called autophagy that cleans out the toxins from your cells. When triggered by intermittent fasting, as well as other methods such as the keto diet and exercise, autophagy slowly gets you habituated into healthier lifestyle habits like, eating nutritious foods and exercising.

This book doesn't skip a beat in telling you how to make intermittent fasting a seamless part of your life. The book even covers topics like how pregnant women and women over 50 can successfully start intermittent fasting. Read on to change how you look and feel for good.

Most people get interested in intermittent fasting and autophagy because of what they can do for their weight and for the natural detox. While these benefits are something you don't want to miss, it is astounding how intermittent fasting can do even more for you. When we talk about the many positive effects intermittent fasting has on your body, we can split them into two categories: effects that you see fairly soon and long-term effects that are even more important in the grand scheme of things.

The effects that you see early on include younger-looking skin with a glow, weight loss, and an increase in the energy you have to spend every day. These alone usually convince people that they should do intermittent fasting to trigger autophagy, but there is even more it can do for them. That's because this advanced process you will see in your body will cause all the operations in your body to run much more smoothly, leading to countless positive effects like less inflammation, lower cholesterol, lowered risk of cancer, lowered risk of heart disease, and a massive reduction in the knots and tangles in the brain linked to neurodegenerative diseases like Alzheimer's disease and Parkinson's disease.

It would be hard to decide which effects to your health you care about more, but fortunately, there is no need for you to choose. If you follow a new routine of intermittent fasting, you will get all of them — and this book has everything you could possibly need to know about how to get there.

There are plenty of books on this subject on the market, thanks again for choosing this one! Every effort was made to ensure it is full of as much useful information as possible; please enjoy!

Chapter 1

The American Woman who Wants to Lose Weight

"The philosophy of fasting calls upon us to know ourselves, to master ourselves, and to discipline ourselves, the better to free ourselves. To fast is to identify our dependencies and free ourselves from them."

- Tariq Ramadan

The desire to lose weight is very common among American women, but it isn't the only thing they want for their bodies. Luckily, intermittent has been proven by research to spur weight loss in American women that were studied, but its health benefits go far beyond weight loss. If you want to feel more energetic, lower your risk of heart disease, and reduce inflammation, intermittent fasting is one lifestyle change that will accomplish all these.

In the four years between 2013 and 2016, half of American citizens said that they wanted to lose weight. This means you are far from the only person in your position, so it isn't surprising that more women that were surveyed said they wanted to drop some pounds. While around 60% of women said they had put effort into losing weight, only about 40% of men said the same. Moreover, age plays into it too: just 40% of adults say that they want to lose weight, while 60% of adults under this age say they do. These results from gender and age go across all other demographics: race, income, education, and so on. It has also been found that the more someone weighs, the more likely it is that they say they want to lose weight.

People who want to lose weight employ all sorts of techniques to achieve this end. First of all, the most commonly seen techniques are dieting and exercise; as we will see in the book, these two techniques are essential to having success in your health and body. Nowhere in this book will I say that you should not be doing these things.

However, there is a mountain of evidence that the best way to make progress in weight loss is the one that these chapters cover: intermittent fasting in order to trigger autophagy. If you don't believe me, we will continue to cite scientific research backing up this claim, and if you need more, you can read through the appendix of studies at the back of the book. The beauty of this technique is that it requires so little change in your day-to-day life when compared to others.

American women have a lot to think about besides losing weight, so a technique that interferes with your life as little as possible is the most practical approach to take. A practical approach like intermittent fasting also makes it more likely that you will continue to follow it through, instead of quitting shortly after starting the way that many women do with diet and exercise. If you make exercise your main technique for losing weight, you have to establish a new routine of going to the gym with relative frequency. Of course, all of us could find time in our schedules to do that, but the issue is that changing our schedules so drastically makes us far less likely to keep on track with it. If diet is your main technique, you run into the same obstacle, so your excitement over dieting fades rather quickly, once you realize all the planning and calorie counting it demands.

As I will elaborate on later, eating right and exercise are both necessary to some extent to achieve an advanced state of this process. They are even more necessary once you get to a certain point in your autophagy journey and become obsessed with triggering it as much as possible, but that will come naturally in the future. For now, you need a plan to slim down that will work reliably. Intermittent fasting is that plan.

The coming chapters will expand on the definition of intermittent fasting, what benefits you can expect to get from it, and what kinds of it may best suit you. In the meantime, you need to have a basic idea of it to work with.

Intermittent fasting is the practice of going between periods eating ("feasting") and not eating ("fasting"). There are a lot of ways this can be done, but a simple way to start is choosing an amount of time that you will fast every day. You can even start with a number as low as 5 hours and work from there.

An American woman who fasts for 5 hours every day could commit herself not to eat between the hours of 1pm and 6pm every day. After around a month has passed and she has found this to work in her routine, she will want to add a few more hours, making it a 7 hour fast. When this one works longer for another month, she can add more hours to it. A reasonable stretch goal to aim for in the beginning is about 10 to 12 hours, even with just one small change in your daily eating routine, you can notice surprising changes to your health and body. That is what makes it such a great way of losing weight and unlocking numerous other positive effects on your body.

A Broad Look at How an American Woman Can Lose Weight with Intermittent Fasting

So far, we have explained the reason why intermittent fasting (often shortened to IF) is the perfect solution for you if you want to make your body look and feel healthier.

But in this book, I don't only want to bring IF and autophagy to the general public's attention. I want to our in-depth review of these phenomenally effective lifestyle changes to reach the American woman in particular.

Thus, if you are an American woman struggling to lose weight, I hope this chapter succeeds in letting you know that *Intermittent Fasting for Women 101* was written for you, especially.

The bulk of our walkthrough on IF is going to be about IF itself. However, as effective as it can surprisingly be on its own, we still have to spend some time discussing diet and exercise, because they can make a large impact, too.

Even with IF on our side, there are general guidelines for losing weight that always apply. For one, a woman trying to slim down will have to take in fewer calories than she is currently, this is just math. A woman who is IF consistently but eating the same number of calories in the narrower window of time is not going to find significant success.

Secondly, you have to eat the right foods, as you could potentially eat fewer calories than you were before but be getting them from all the wrong places: sugar, saturated fats, and intermittent fasting's biggest enemy, the carbs. Instead, you should get your calories from foods that have plenty of important nutrients, vitamins, and minerals. These are foods like fatty fish, whole grains low in carbs, nuts, non-starchy vegetables, some fruit, leafy greens, and more.

We will have plenty of space to go in more detail on which foods to eat in our chapter dedicated to that specifically, but this is your essential aliment. Essentially, you want to think about what is really in your food from the standpoint of nutrients. Besides, you want to think about how the foods you consume will really affect your body, and once you get used to it, eating healthily is not as cumbersome as you think.

The little things are what matter when it comes to your body and health. For this reason, we still have to dive into the basics of weight loss, despite IF being such a reliable method. The first little thing is eating these nutrient-rich foods instead of the nutrient-poor calorie-rich foods you may be used to. The second little thing is getting more exercise. Most American women say they reach their weight goals the most when they follow a consistent routine of diet and exercise, but you should keep in mind that your diet will be more efficient than exercise.

Your doctor can help you along your journey to lose weight and answer specific questions that we may not be able to specifically address here. In case you don't visit the doctor soon, you will probably hear the following advice from them: (1) follow the two little things above, (2) get enough sleep every night, and (3) control your level of stress. I do recommend you talk to a doctor when making a lifestyle change like following IF, though. Healthy people can make this routine without issue the vast majority of the time, but talking to a doctor about it can put you at ease.

You are probably cognizant of the fact that different people can use the same methods to lose weight and get very different results. Genes are not the only thing playing a role, though. Everyone burns some calories even when they are not exercising, but the rate at which the calories burn depends on your DNA, the current state of your anatomy, and your health history.

It might help you to keep track of your calories, but perhaps even more important is keeping track of where your calories are coming from. For example, are they coming from nutrient-rich sources, or from calorie-rich, nutrient-poor sources? One of them will help you lose weight, and the other damage you.

Now we need to discuss the matter of how many calories you take in. Logically, you will, of course, lose more weight the fewer calories you consume, but that is not a good thing if you don't eat enough. Doctors say that a woman eating fewer than around 900 calories will hurt you more than help you. Eating fewer calories every day will certainly help you reach your weight goal, but you have to make sure you do it the right way. Not getting enough energy will not only harm your body, but it will not ultimately help you lose weight anyway. If you faint from lack of energy sources, you will lose your self-control and eat a lot in order to get your energy back up, and this will put you back where you started.

As the saying goes, slow and steady wins the race. So, you should limit your calories at a steady, reasonable amount. By simply consuming as few calories as possible will not help you at all in the long run, as it can be tempting when you desperately want to drop several pounds at once, but I strongly urge you not to do this. You can speak with your doctor about how many calories you can safely reduce your daily consumption without running into any health risks. The number they will give you depends on your height, current weight, age, and level of activity.

American women often ask the question: are men better able to lose weight than women? The answer is

138

complicated. It can seem like men have an easier time dropping weight than women, but you have to remember that there are several factors involved: women tend to have a greater share of fat on their bodies compared to muscle, while men tend to have more muscle compared to fat. Since muscle burns more calories than fat, this may be part of the reason that they seem to have an easier time than women.

When you eat, you are in part giving nutrients to your muscles. Men have more muscle on average, so when they eat, more of their calories go to support their muscle. Women, on the other hand, don't have as much muscle to support, so less of their calorie consumption will have this job, and instead, it is more likely to be stored as fat.

Now, I tell everyone, man or woman, that they should try intermittent fasting if they want to lose weight. That said, there are reasons that this works out for women in particular. For instance, one experiment had one group of women losing weight by avoiding unhealthy food, while the other group tried to lose weight by lowering their consumption of calories overall by eating smaller portions. The end result was that the group of women eating fewer calories overall had lower BMIs (body mass indices), by the end of the study.

The same experiment was done on men, and the results were not as strong for them. This suggests that while limiting calories consumed overall could be a better option for women, the kinds of foods consumed may be more important to focus on for men.

As usual, I want to clarify that the specific foods you eat are still very important. Bringing out this scientific study was only meant to serve the purpose of telling you what is vital.

American women should put foods in their bodies that contain the nutrients they need and exercise, but when your main goal is losing weight, the thing you want to focus on most of all is the number of calories consumed. As long as you keep this number at a safe level, you will optimize your success with IF and autophagy.

This is where yet another advantage of IF comes into play. The gains you have from it are partially from the simple fact of consuming fewer calories. When you don't eat at all during a certain window of the day, this ends up reducing your total number of calories consumed per day. That benefit is only one positive effect of intermittent fasting, although it is a terrific benefit. The most important benefits come from the autophagy triggered by IF. We will have a lot to learn about this process in the early chapters.

But on the subject of how an American woman can lose weight, there is still much to consider. We have not even gotten to managing your menstrual cycle while losing weight; being on your period doesn't make your weight go up or down, so it can influence your weight in indirect ways. Consequently, you will have more of an appetite for sugary and salty food when you have PMS (premenstrual syndrome), as one example. Obviously, eating more foods like these can have quite an effect on your weight, even though your cycle doesn't affect your mass directly. The higher levels of salt in your body can even make your system soak up more water instead of disposing of it, giving you more water weight. These ways that your cycle makes losing weight harder can be especially troublesome as an American woman, where sugary and salty foods are widespread and cheap. Your best bet for resisting these temptations is not buying them in the first place, so fill your pantry and fridge with nutrient-rich foods, and don't put the sugary and salty foods there to begin with.

The same way your period can indirectly affect your weight, your weight can affect your period as well. Although our end goal is to slim down, losing weight or gaining weight in a short span of time can have consequences for your menstrual cycle, as your period may not come on time or may not come at all. Many women with weight problems like obesity have this issue. On the other hand, if your period is coming on schedule on a regular basis, this is a good indicator of overall health. Accomplishing your goal weight will help make your period come at a regular schedule.

Trying to lose weight can also become a challenge after menopause. For example, on average menopausal women put on 5 pounds. Estrogen actually helps regulate your weight, so the fact that your estrogen levels are lower may be part of the reason it is harder to lose weight or maintain it. But we can't only blame it on menopause. Oftentimes, gaining mass at this stage in life can be due to a slowed metabolism that comes with age in general, eating too many unhealthy foods and not enough healthy ones, and not getting enough exercise.

We also lose significant muscle mass with age. With less muscle mass comes fewer calories than our bodies use, and therefore convert to fat. All of these facts about losing weight on menopause should teach us to do the same two little things that all American women should do: keep up an active lifestyle and eat healthful foods.

If you are an American woman over the age of 50, I also recommend that you don't eat as many calories that you used to when you were younger. There are two main reasons for this: (1) women don't need as many calories as men because of having less muscle mass, more fat, and being smaller in size in general, and (2) women over 50 tend to expend less energy than they used to, so they don't need as many calories in the first place.

If you fall into the demographic of women over 50, you should speak with your doctor about how many calories you can safely limit your diet to lose weight. Their answer may surprise you because women generally don't need as many calories when they are older.

Intermittent Fasting as an Alternative to Less Healthy Methods that May Not Even Work

When American women try to slim down, they have many options with which to approach the situation. Unfortunately, many of them will only help you lose weight that you will put back on the moment you get back into your normal routine. Not only that, but they can have negative health consequences.

It is astonishing how many doctors now recommend weight-loss prescriptions to menopausal women. Usually, they will only do this if you have a BMI over 30 (if you are obese) or if you are overweight and you are looking at other health risks because of your weight as determined by hypertension or high cholesterol. Additionally, a good doctor will make sure you have tried the two little things we mentioned earlier before prescribing you medicine: regular exercise and dieting. They will normally only prescribe it to you if you do not see results from these methods. While it is understandable to want to avoid the health risks of being overweight or obese, the side effects that accompany these medicines may outweigh the benefits. They include migraines, coughing, tiredness, constipation, and even dissociation.

Again, it makes complete sense that a doctor might prescribe these medications to women so they can lose mass and can be at lower risk for diseases related to weight. But it is not necessary for you to take these measures and accept these side effects, because you can do intermittent fasting instead. IF has no side effects — only good ones, like triggering autophagy and losing weight. Much like taking a pill, IF doesn't require much change in your daily life. It only requires that you *don't* do something during a small window of your day: eat.

Many American women are choosing this method over medication because of it: you can join them today. These upcoming chapters equip you with all the information you need to do IF successfully so you can enjoy its effects on your body and health.

Chapter 2

What is Intermittent Fasting?

"The best of all medicines is resting and fasting."

- Benjamin Franklin

Fasting has become a hot topic as of late. The buzz around intermittent fasting, in particular, opened a door for many women who wanted to lose weight but were worried about the heavy commitment of a day-long water-only fast. It's hard to say exactly what IF is because there are a variety of ways to go about it. When you do an intermittent fast, you are going back and forth in a regular cycle between fasting and eating normally. I will cover all types of it in this book, and you can decide which best suits your stage in life and goals.

Many women have seen real change happen in their health, thanks to IF. You could join them by following the various tips contained here. The first task we have to complete is giving you a broad overview of all things: what the benefits are, what the science says, what different kinds of intermittent fasting exist, and what foods you should eat.

We can start with the health benefits. Women who follow this kind of routine feel that they have more energy, burn more fat, and lower their chances of getting diabetes or heart disease. Researchers looking into IF find that its practitioners have higher success rates than people who do extended, interrupted fasts and people who use exercise as their chief method to lose weight. Thus, they suggest the success of IF it can be woven seamlessly into the participants' lives without their having to change multiple aspects of their normal routines.

Furthermore, it eliminates the perfectionism that sometimes ruins other weight loss techniques. It doesn't ask that you constantly pay attention to the number of calories you consume and it doesn't punish you harshly for falling out of it for one day.

145

We will learn more about the science underlying IF later on but suffice to say that you can earn the positive health effects of autophagy without doing extended fasts. The experiments studying people doing IF consistently demonstrate that they see good results from only doing it, without doing more demanding fasts such as extended water fasting.

In the last chapter, we talked about the study showing that women have more success in losing weight by reducing caloric intake compared to when they pay close attention to what they are eating. This is precisely what IF entails. Nutrition is still important, which is why we still have a chapter on it, but regardless of what you eat, you will still see some amount of positive change from IF.

I hope that I have at least made you curious about getting these results from IF in your own life — and to do that, you will need to find a way to implement IF in a way that works for you. It's time to answer the question directly: in the simplest terms, what do I have to do to start with it today? What is required of me to start seeing these effects on my health?

Because of the nature of this process, you will, unfortunately, have to start tomorrow, not today — unless it is morning right now. Ask yourself how many hours you think you can fast tomorrow. Let's say it is 6 hours. Most people start their fast after lunch and break it for dinner. Keep in mind that you will have to eat lunch relatively early so that you do not have dinner too late. If you have dinner too late, your system will take hours to start up autophagy while you sleep because you will still be digesting food. You should be able to see now why many women find they are able to succeed in losing weight when they were not successful using other methods. What I described in the last paragraph is all that IF amounts to on your end.

Of course, practice is always harder than theory. I will never tell you that intermittent fasting takes no willpower and resistance on your end. Compared to other potential options, though, it is extremely straightforward. Still, you might have a long way to go to be ready to live by it. Maybe you still need to be convinced by the number of studies that we will cover proving the health benefits. Maybe you are scientifically minded and need to learn more about autophagy.

You might get inspired when I tell you all the delicious foods you can eat when you intermittent fast to make autophagy even stronger; you might be ready to start after you read about all the different kinds of IF, and you find the one that is perfect for you.

The chapters after this one will explore these topics and more. This one will give you a general idea of all of them so you can keep reading with an informed picture of what you are getting into. You may even choose to check the Table of Contents and read the chapters that interest you the most first. It is your choice, just be sure to read through all of them at some point, so you don't miss any important knowledge.

Intermittent Fasting: Looking at its Effects on Health More Closely

In few words, it helps you slim down using short-term and long-term strategies, by depriving your system of calories so you accumulate less fat in the short term and by detoxifying your cells in the long term through a process, the autophagy. The short-term strategy is what tends to draw women in, but the long-term strategy is what makes IF great for your body overall.

This is not the same kind of detox that you may be sick of hearing about online. The autophagy triggered by IF is a detox that has always existed in biology and can simply be jumpstarted naturally by fasting. While a detox like "juicing" will claim to clean out your system, supporters of juice diets have no data to back up this assertion. Meanwhile, the process has been studied by scientists and nutritionists for decades now. We know that it works to lose weight. We know that it does so without hurting your body the way that other methods do — not only does it not hurt your body, but it has long-term positive consequences like less inflammation and lower cholesterol.

Every organism on the planet goes through it, so you are not even putting your body through anything strange to get these effects on your health. If you had never heard of the word 'autophagy' before, it would still occur in your body. By learning how to trigger it through intermittent fasting, you are simply learning how to optimize it. This procedure doesn't involve any strange medicines or foods. Whatever you put into your body; you can still trigger it with IF.

Of course, your diet does affect how powerful your autophagy is, but we will talk about that in a moment. For now, I want to tell you more about the short-term effects of IF. The first we will explore is the enhanced health of your skin. The first layer of skin that you have is called the epidermis; you see your epidermis every day because this is the visible part of your skin. There are layers of skin below it, but you don't see those layers unless you suffer an injury. We will go into more scientific detail on this process in the section after this one, but you will need a crash course to understand why it is triggered by IF is so good for your skin, and your epidermis in specific.

Both parts of the English word "autophagy" are of Greek origin. "Auto" has the meaning "self" (which you might already know) and "phagy" has the meaning "eat." Put the two together, and you get the fundamental concept of autophagy. Therefore, your cells "eat themselves" when they are under acute stress. Unlike you, your cells need energy constantly — even when you are sleeping, they will get it from whatever source they can find. Even when you are not putting food into your body (even when you are fasting), your cells find ways of getting energy. When in this state of stress, their main sources of energy are the following: cell organelles that stopped working, proteins that are no longer being used, and toxins that came from outside your body.

For your first fast, you will notice big changes in your body after only a day. These drastic changes are thanks to this method. I guarantee you the first change you will notice is in your skin; it will remind you of when you were younger because of its newfound elasticity and glow, so these improvements in your skin are because of it. Besides, on an invisible level of your skin pores, your skin cells are cleaning out the toxins described above. On the massive scale of your whole pore, that makes a huge difference. The autophagy results in skin that isn't filled with cellular waste.

The cleaning out of cellular waste isn't the only reason your skin gets better. It's also because you have an increase in the collagen protein in your skin. Collagen is a protein that your skin cells make more of when you are younger and is the reason the skin of younger people looks the way it is. As you get older, your skin cells make less collagen because they are less effective. This is where autophagy changes everything. Sure enough, it does two things to make new, young cells: (1) builds them from scratch using the raw materials obtained from eating their own cellular waste or (2) renovates existing cells with new organelles constructed with raw materials obtained from eating their own cellular waste.

Everything should be coming together with IF and autophagy now. It all goes like this: you do even a moderate level of fasting that increases your autophagy and then when your skin cells go through it, they make younger cells or make existing cells like younger cells.

The best part is that the improved health of your skin is only the beginning. The main reason everyone who does IF does it is because they want to lose weight. Fasting proves time and time again that it is the best way of doing it. This point has already been driven home, so I will add just one extra point to it: you won't just lose weight, but you will be able to relax about loose skin as well.

The infamous "skin curtain" is the excess skin that people are afraid of getting when they lose weight. It is astonishing how many people say they don't want to lose weight out of fear of loose skin. However, the good news is that this process comes to the rescue on this front. By losing weight through fasting, you cut down on calories and trigger autophagy at the same time. Thus, its job is to break down poorly performing cells and replace them with new, young cells, or at least replace their organelles with new ones. That's why people who lose weight through fasting are proven to deal with far fewer issues with loose skin. Not only do they have less loose skin to deal with in the beginning, but they are better able to manage what loose skin they do have because of the better health of their skin.

I told you that you would have more energy when you did IF, and now it's time to explain the scientific reason why. Autophagy is behind it, as usual and maybe you have already deduced why by now. The short answer is that the autophagy that IF triggers makes your cells more efficient, and more efficient cells means more energy for you.

As you get older, your cells are less effective than they used to be. They are littered with cellular waste and their cell organs (organelles) are damaged and ineffective in themselves. Autophagy is the remedy to this problem: it disposes of organelles that aren't performing optimally and disposes of cellular waste and misfolded proteins that are taking up space in your cells without doing anything useful. When all of your cells go through it regularly and take care of these issues, you have more energy because your cells make up all of you, and that makes your system more efficient with energy overall.

Now let's go in more detail on the long-term positive health effects.

There is research showing that this mechanism will fight against tumors, and there is also research showing that it will help them grow — only because cancer cells are cells, too. Although it can work on both sides, the important thing is that it promotes the health of your non-cancerous cells, which will always outnumber your cancerous ones in the early stages. Of course, most people triggering autophagy are doing it to prevent cancer in the early stages and not to stop cancer that is already progressing, so this is all they need. Intermittent fasting has been found to be a powerful tool in combating cancer, while cancer, in general, is still under debate as something that autophagy can prevent altogether, the jury is no longer out for Alzheimer's disease, Parkinson's disease, and Huntington's Disease. Furthermore, this mechanism has been proven to be incredibly effective for matters of the brain.

For long-term problems especially, it is a powerful tool for ensuring the viability and survivability of cells. Scientists did not see it as such a big actor for these diseases until recently. This discovery changes everything scientists thought they knew about the biological process. Excitingly, as I keep telling you, you can trigger it yourself through IF.

But cancer is far from the only age-related condition that autophagy can address: diseases of the mind, heart disease, diseases related to autoimmune failure, and more can be helped with it. While we still aren't sure if this can stop tumors from continuing to grow altogether once they reach a certain size, we know that they can keep the rest of your body around the tumor healthy. This can only be a good thing for fighting cancer, and it's why it is useful in preventing all these other diseases too.

In diabetic people, there are clusters of protein built up in their arteries. Thanks to the two processes working together, scientists can see that these protein clusters are cleared out.

Sometimes books about the newest findings in science with regard to health can be misleading about what the scientific consensus is, but I want this one to be clear about what all scientists agree on. This way, it is as useful and truthful to women as possible.

We know for sure it is a main player — if not *the* main player — in fighting against neurodegenerative diseases like Huntington's, Alzheimer's, and Parkinson's, as it plays this role by cleaning out the build-ups of proteins that happen in your neurons, leading to clogging and brain dysfunction.

Scientists even agree about what causes these protein buildups in the first place, at this point. As your autophagy occurs in the brain, a special organelle called the autophagosome binds with your lysosome (your cell stomach). In many cases of it, this is the normal way that it occurs. Your autophagosome binds with your lysosome in order to break down the cellular waste.

However, what causes the protein buildups is the abnormally strong bond that the autophagosome has with the lysosome. This strong bond between the autophagosome and the lysosome causes what biologists call a "clogging effect." The clogging effect makes your proteins build up in your neurons, leading to neurodegeneration.

You can read more about the details of this science soon enough, but these are the basics of what causes these diseases. As you can see, this process is at the very center of it. If you want to prevent these diseases — as everyone does — you have to trigger it as much as possible, so your cells clean out your proteins.

You might think this sounds counterintuitive since these buildups happen in the first place because of autophagy occurring and the autophagosome binding too tightly with the lysosome, but this abnormal binding is only an issue when your autophagy is occurring at a maintenance level. Scientists who study it say that yours is in "maintenance mode" when it is happening at a low level, just as it always does. You see, this is always happening in your body somewhere, but that does not mean it is happening at a significant level.

Your autophagosome and lysosome can cause the "clogging effect" when your autophagy only happens in maintenance mode and you do not trigger the advanced one to clean out the resulting protein buildup. All you have to do to clear out this protein build up is do intermittent fasting, trigger the advanced one, and prevent the protein buildup that could cause you to go through neurodegeneration. If you want to know more about the biology of this process or about the link between neurodegenerative diseases and autophagy, you will have plenty to look forward to in the coming chapters. For now, we will continue outlining the long-term benefits of both of them.

We listed losing weight as a short-term effect, which it is — but it is also a long-term benefit. People who are overweight or obese have higher risk of heart disease, diabetes, and failing autoimmune systems. When you lose weight, you lower your risk of all these problems.

Therefore, you should also consider it to have a long-term positive effect on your health.

While this won't apply to every woman's situation, there has also been testing on the effects of autophagy on people going through chemotherapy for cancer. The researchers looked at a group going through therapy without fasting and a group who did IF during the chemotherapy.

The group that fasted while going through chemotherapy had significantly lower amounts of dead white blood cells in their systems. If you don't know already, chemotherapy has some negative side effects when it kills cancer cells, and one of them is killing good cells like white blood cells.

White blood cells do a very important job when they are alive, but like every other cell, they become toxic when they die. Unfortunately, chemotherapy tends to kill a lot of white blood cells in the process of killing cancer cells.

That's where the method comes in. The patients who fasted during chemotherapy had significantly less dead white blood cells creating toxins in their bodies because intermittent fasting got rid of them. IF led their bodies to seek nutrients from inside the body; there were a lot of dead white blood cells in their body, so autophagy took care of those. As a result, they did not have all these dead cells polluting their bodies.

There is a lot of research about the effect of autophagy triggered by fasting on people with cancer. Another study looked at women with breast cancer who did a fast lasting 12 hours daily. These women did not see their cancer return as often as women who did not fast. This means that not only it does have implications for lessening the side effects of common cancer treatment likes chemotherapy, but it can even lower the chances that your cancer will come back once it goes.

We are still waiting to see if pharmacists can manage to create a medicine that will take advantage of the power of this mechanism. There are supplements that claim to trigger it, but none of those claims are substantial at the moment, so your best option is to focus on making it happen through intermittent fasting. But it is possible that, one day, scientists will use their knowledge on it to create a medicine that cures diseases like Alzheimer's and cancer. Thus, the possibilities are endless.

As far as long-term benefits of autophagy go, it has even been shown to lower the amount of inflammation in your body. When you have less inflammation in your body, your DNA in your cells is far less likely to be damaged. Damaged DNA and high inflammation are big risk factors for diseases like cancer, so these are highly important long-term effects. Whereas parts of your body are inflamed, it does its part by taking care of these damages. Once these damages have been taken care of, you can make new parts that are newer, younger, and less vulnerable to damage. It has even been shown that mice who were bred in a lab who went through autophagy triggered through fasting had lower rates of cancer than rats who did not fast. The ones who did not trigger it had higher rates of cancer.

Your digestive health is surprisingly important to your long-term health outcomes, and it can help in keeping this part of your body healthy as well. It is so important because the parts of your body that control your digestive system are constantly working — they never stop. When they give your digestive system a break by fasting, you are giving it time to stop what it is doing and do repairs. Your tissues in your digestive system have the opportunity to clear out cellular waste and make their systems more efficient at the cellular level.

This makes this system of your body more efficient, all because you are able to trigger autophagy to keep it clean. People often underestimate the importance of their gut health, but it is actually one of the parts of your body you should protect the most. If you are not able to get nutrients with a healthy gut, none of the other systems in your body are able to work the way they should.

We would be remiss to forget about your autoimmune system in the context of autophagy. Your autoimmune system is the way your body attack infections and disease, as it fights cancer before it can grow to the size of a tumor. But it isn't only about cancer: your autoimmune system keeps any infection from turning into a disease.

Doctors now say that preventive medicine is the most important kind of medicine, and your autoimmune system is the main player in your body's natural disease preventive mechanism. While you do intermittent fasting, you keep this vital system healthy and prevent age-related disease. So, this is a good place to start when describing all the good things autophagy can do for your body by simply limiting the window of time that you are eating every day. However, if you want to get the short-term and long-term effects, you have to keep a few things in mind.

First of all, you can't expect to get these results by simply fasting every once in a while. If you eat poorly, drink a lot, smoke, get little sleep, or have any number of habits that are bad for your health, you can't expect to do IF and have it repair all the damage you do to your body from these habits. Successfully triggering autophagy with intermittent fasting requires that you are at least somewhat healthy in other areas of your habits as well; the first needs your body to maintain some level of basic health in order to do its job. It can't do that job without your help.

There is not enough space in this book to tell you how to stop all of these bad habits, but I will do our best to consider the lifestyle of the average American woman when helping you get IF into your life.

Intermittent Fasting and Autophagy

Autophagy is the natural way your body disposes of toxic chemicals in your cells; you can't see it happening without a microscope, but your cells have been going through it for your entire life without you ever noticing. In just the last twenty years, scientists have learned much about the metabolic its process. Most importantly for our purposes, they have learned more and more about how its implications for fighting against disease and aging.

The entire foundation of using IF for losing weight and getting healthier is our current scientific understanding of autophagy. We know for a fact that it can help us attain better general health and live longer. So, it isn't just for losing weight, however — although it does that job better than any other method. It used to be that people went through this process quite often. We went through it more back in the days before industrial agriculture because we did not expect to have food all the time.

Nowadays in the industrialized world, most people rarely miss a meal. We always have food around us, but people back in the day did not even have an expectation to eat every single day. Our bodies went through advanced autophagy very regularly because of this and we can even say that our bodies are more built for not eating every day than they are for eating constantly as we do right now.

Our first encounter with this mechanism in the world of science was thanks to the French scientist named Christian De Duve. He and a group of biologists took note of a bizarre organelle that they had never seen before; they named it the lysosome.

Scientists thought that the lysosome was simply an organelle made for disposing of garbage. If you think about it, this doesn't even make logical sense, because there is not really such thing as disposing of something. You can change the form of something, but not dispose of it. If the lysosome was really an organelle that just kept breaking things down without recycling those parts, then eventually those tiny waste particles would build-up with nowhere to go.

Now we have an explanation for this problem because of autophagy, and this explanation has important takeaways for doctors, biologists, and anyone who cares about their health.

The Japanese scientist Yoshinori Ohsumi was the first scientist to get deeply interested in the lysosome of yeast cells. 2016 was the year he won the Nobel Prize when he learned that the lysosome was the center of a cellular process called autophagy. His key finding was that our cells never "dispose of" anything — they simply break down cellular waste into raw materials, and then use these materials to build new structures.

Ohsumi has created a new definition of this process. He says that it is the way our cells break down waste materials for the purpose of freeing up space, killing harmful foreign toxins, and creating raw materials that can be used for building new cells. When Ohsumi first started, he was the first scientist to really have any interest in this topic. He started a scientific movement around it when his research uncovered all the implications that autophagy has for our bodies. Not only did Ohsumi uncover much of our modern understanding of autophagy, but he was the one who coined the phrase "cell recycling." Cell recycling is what happens once autophagy is finished.

When your cells have cleaned themselves out, they use these raw materials for constructing things that other cells can use. They can also use these raw materials to create new cells if there is enough.

Now we know that this can be considered the most important process for your cells both individually and collectively; it matters to your cells individually because it keeps them alive as well as possible; it matters collectively because your cells have to work together to be useful to your body as a whole, and it keeps them working together smoothly when the process keeps them repaired and "cleaned out."

We will have an entire chapter dedicated to the science that makes intermittent fasting such a great way of keeping your system in great shape. For now, this should provide you with all you need to know to continue on with a solid understanding of the underlying process of autophagy making your fasting worth it.

You also need to keep in mind the times that you should be eating these foods. The whole purpose of this process is lost if you eat during the times you are supposed to fast. That's because consuming anything puts your digestive system at work. When your body digests food, your autophagy stops. You need to really make sure you are not eating at all during these times that you have designated to be your fasting windows.

Even eating 20 calories disrupts autophagy entirely. You may think that eating a banana or a small snack during your fasting window won't change anything, but that isn't true at all. You would be shocked at how much changes in your body when you put food into it. The fact that so much changes is the reason why it is so potent in the first place — because it is recovering from all the times that you were putting food into your body.

The Ideal Diet for a Woman Doing Intermittent Fasting

Before we dive into the subject of what you eat when you fast, I need to issue a warning to you: there are people selling supplements that they say will trigger autophagy. At the moment, no such supplements exist. That means you need to be wary of claims like these. There are scientists trying to create a medication with this effect, but it has not been made yet.

The first important vitamin is also the easiest one to get into your body: Vitamin D. This is an essential vitamin to a myriad of biological processes that your system goes through, and autophagy is one of them — so if you don't have enough Vitamin D, you won't be able to get the one that you need.

You don't ever want to think about diet as your only means of triggering autophagy. Everything needs to be in place to some extent: you need to keep up a diet of nutrient-rich foods, exercise, get plenty of sleep, avoid unhealthy habits, and fast. The great thing about it is that it focuses certain organs in your body to make sure you are getting it where you need it.

We will start with ginger as an example to illustrate this. Ginger contains a chemical called 6-shogaol, which actually slows the growth of cells in your lungs. It probably seems counterproductive to ingest something that stops your cells from growing when you are trying to prevent cancer or some other lung disease. However, ginger is an excellent complement to autophagy because this chemical suppresses cell growth.

6-shogaol suppresses all cell growth, meaning that even cancer cells will not be able to grow as well when you add this chemical into your system.

Omega-3 fats are probably something that you have heard of before. They are considered a "healthy fat," a kind of fat that your body needs. People who get plenty of these healthy fats into their bodies have been shown to have more advanced autophagy than people who do not. So, it is greatly aided by unsaturated fats like Omega-3 fats.

With that in mind, you should know that with Omega-3 fats and all of the nutrients we mention, you need to make a real effort to get them from your regular diet rather than from supplements. For example, the effectiveness of Omega-3 fats in making people's bodies healthier and supporting autophagy are scientifically substantiated, but it has only been tested in people who got them from real food like fish. There is no backing to the idea that the Omega-3 fats that some people get some supplements are going to give you this same effect.

Getting your Omega-3 fats from a supermarket is not your best option, either. Grocery stores these days are known to get their meats from factory farms. Meat coming from factory farms does not have Omega-3 fats because of what factory farms feed their cattle. Instead of eating grass or other natural foods, they consume a lot of chemicals. Instead of indirectly getting the Omega-3 fats from grass through your meat, you are indirectly getting whatever chemical foods these factory farms give to their animals.

It goes without saying that you need to eat plenty of vegetables when you are doing intermittent fasting, too. It is a simple fact that a lot of people don't like vegetables at all, but thankfully there are ways of getting around this. One of them is putting your vegetables in a blender together with some fruit. If you get your vegetables this way, you should remember not to add too much fruit into the blender. While fruits are good for us, they have a lot of natural sugar in them, which is still bad for us in large quantities just like artificial sugars.

The next thing you should consider consuming to help the two processes is green tea. The chemical in green tea that you are really looking for triggers AMPK, which is an enzyme in your system that boosts the effectiveness of autophagy. Lastly, Green tea goes best with turmeric, because they both help.

Next, you should find somewhere that you can start picking up the reishi mushroom and eating it on the regular. The reishi mushroom is a special case because it can significantly slow the growth of one cell in particular: cancer cells in the colon. The colon is a very common place to start seeing cancer, so this food is really something that you should consider adding to your diet. It works by helping the growth of non-cancer cells when cancer cells are growing in the colon. When non-cancer cells are able to grow and flourish in your body alongside cancer cells, this really helps keep cancer at bay and fight it. Each cell does its part in trying to overwhelm the cancer cells. Normally, the cancer cells in the colon will actively try to stop the non-cancer cells from growing, and the chemicals in the reishi mushroom does their part in keeping this from occurring.

Looking at autophagy and intermittent fasting from the perspective of diet can be very inspiring because you can look at them from more than one point of view. You feel as though you are triggering autophagy in every way possible from the simple action of eating certain foods that you know for sure are helpful.

Good practitioners of these two mechanisms will use several methods to make their autophagy as strong as possible. I have done extensive research about what scientists say on these different diets, and I am only recommending foods to you that are proved to work.

If you are still having issues deciding which approach is right for you, looking at the foods you eat might be a good place to start. This book strongly recommends IF since it is known to be the most consistent way of getting more autophagy to happen in your system, but everyone is different, so you might want to think about all of your options.

You also need to think about what not to eat when you are thinking about autophagy. Our number one enemy against it is carbs. Everyone knows about the bad reputation that carbs have, but not enough know exactly why we should lessen how many carbs we put into our bodies. Did you know that the average American gets nearly 60% of their calories every day from carbs? It seems incredible, but it's true. Not only do American women have the issue of eating a lot of calories without a plan to burn them off with exercise, but they are getting many of these calories from a source that is notoriously difficult for your system to break down.

Here is the true reason that makes carbs so dangerous, especially for someone who has a plan to do IF: when your gut is holding all of your foods and breaking them down, it has proteins, fats, and carbohydrates. No matter how much fat and protein it has to break down, no matter what other factors are at play, your body will always break down carbs first.

This is because the very nature of carbohydrates makes them extremely challenging to break down. Therefore, your stomach will decide to work on them last. This is why you need to choose a diet that is very low in carbs if you want to succeed in intermittent fasting. Your new life as a slimmer, healthier, and more youthful woman may even

165

depend upon you eating fewer carbs. You will be surprised how many times a day carbs make their way into your diet. This will seriously impair your autophagy. Another way of illustrating this is by looking at how much it reduces it.

We can use an example where you finish eating a meal at 1pm and then stop eating until 9pm. This seems like an 8-hour fast. However, it really is a 4-hour fast; this is because when you stop eating at 1pm, it takes your body 4 hours to digest your food. You aren't done digesting it until 5pm, and then you start eating again at 9pm. Thus, your fast was really 4 hours long. Now, let's put carbohydrates into the picture. Let's say the last meal you eat before you start fasting is a bowl filled with pasta at 1pm, then you don't eat again until 9pm. Take a guess at how long of a fast this really was.

The answer is 0 hours. That's right: it takes 8 hours for your body to digest carbs. Even though you stop eating for 8 hours after the bowl of pasta, your stomach is just now finishing digesting the carbs from the pasta at 9pm, and then you are just putting more food into your body again, stopping autophagy. The latter depends heavily on what you are consuming, it relies on you getting plenty of healthy fats and not eating too many carbs. Practically speaking, most people doing IF to lose weight should reduce their consumption of carbs to be as low as possible.

Now, we need to spend some time talking about fats. It can be confusing because a lot of people are under the impression that fats are bad overall. They don't realize how much their bodies rely on fats to perform basic functions — including autophagy. Not all fats are the

166

same, however. Because of the chemical composition of different fats, some of them are essential, while some of them should be limited to being eaten as little as possible. The fats in your diet can be the hardest thing for you to control, and the way it works can be hard to understand. They can be some of the best things for your body and some of the worst things for your body. First, we will get into what can make them good when you eat the right ones.

Firstly, your system depends on fats because they are one of its sources of energy. Fats can even store vitamins and minerals. Fats are essential for building membranes around your cells and sheaths around your nerves. On a bigger scale, you have fat for moving your muscles, clotting your blood, and keeping your inflammation at normal levels. Generally, we can say that your saturated fats are bad for you, and your unsaturated fats are good for you. Trans fats are especially bad for you, but you don't have to think about that too much, because now they are banned in most places.

Trans fats are a great demonstration of what can make your fats bad. These kinds of fats only come into being because of the industrial, artificial processes that create and preserve food these days. They have no use in your body and can only harm you. This is the reason that they are not allowed in the United States anymore.

Then you have saturated fats. Doctors say that you should be keeping your level of saturated fats to less than 10 percent of all your calories. If at all possible, don't eat saturated fats when you have them as an option.

Meanwhile, doctors want us to get about 30 percent of our calories from good fats. To a lot of people, this seems like a lot of fats for doctors to recommend to us! It goes to show you how different kinds of fats have such different effects on our bodies.

We have plenty more to discuss in the chapter coming later about what foods to eat when doing IF, but this should give you a good preview on what to expect later. Now you can read about what different options you have for methods of IF.

Your Options for Different Methods of Intermittent Fasting

If none of the methods of intermittent fasting discussed thus far appeal to you, this is a section that *will* appeal to you. We will discuss these methods more and hopefully convince you that there is one that suits your needs.

I will start by telling you that IF is by far the most popular way to fast overall. Outside of it, the only other legitimate option is called extended water fasting. Extended water fasting, usually just called water fasting, is when you only consume water for a period of time, usually lasting 24 hours or longer. We will get into it a little bit in this book, but there are many reasons that we will mostly stick to intermittent fasting.

I say that the non-intermittent fasts outside of water fasting are not legitimate simply because there is no research supporting their claims the way there is for both of them. We will start by talking about what other fasts you may hear about, and I will tell you why you can forget about them entirely, because either they won't work to help you lose weight, they are bad for your body, or oftentimes, both. The most dangerous one is called dry fasting. Dry fasting is the same thing as water fasting, but you don't even consume water. It is hard to say why this idea even exists because there is no reason to believe that it would be more effective in helping you lose weight than water fasting. Sure, you will lose water weight for a temporary span of time, but then you will go back to drinking water and gain it all back again. It does not even keep the water weight off of you.

But all of that is beside the point; you don't want to lose water weight. Hydration is one of the most important things to be mindful of when caring for your body, and when it gets too low, that is bad for you in general — not to mention bad for your autophagy. I said to watch your diet, exercise, fasting, and sleep when you want to trigger it, but you have to watch your water consumption, too. Not having any water for your cells dries them out and prevents them from working the way that they should.

Once you get a grip on the intermittent fasting stuff, you might want to dip your toes into water fasting. The best way to do this is by participating in the 24-hour fast.

When you do a true, traditional fast, you don't eat at all for at least a day. This is the essence of the water fast, too, but extended this process can last for multiple days. With the 24-hour fast, you are only dedicating yourself to fasting for 24 hours. This is a lot easier than you might think.

Next, we have what is known as consecutive day fasting. Maybe fasting for a set number of hours every single day sounds like a commitment that you won't be able to keep up. If that's the case, consecutive day fasting might be right for you. You might decide on fasting for 12 hours every other day instead of 8 hours every single day. This way, your fasts balance each other out. Another advantage of the consecutive day fast is you have something to look forward to on your fasting days. You know that you will not have to abstain the next day; this can be very motivating for a lot of people.

When it comes to fasts that you should avoid, we could talk about protein fasting. Protein fasting is when protein is the only thing that you consume. Protein may be an important thing for you to get into your system, but it is definitely not wise to make it the only nutrient you get. In fact, it is best for you to eat a pretty low amount of it. Your body will break down fat before protein, and as a result, your autophagy will be better if you don't eat as much of it. The logic behind this method simply doesn't hold up, so you shouldn't pay any attention to it.

In truth, at the end of the day, this is your body that we are talking about, so the way you choose to fast is your decision alone. You will always have the freedom to tailor your fast any way you want. As long as you follow the guidance in our book, you can do fasting your own way.

Chapter 3:

Benefits of Intermittent Fasting

There is no longer a debate on this point: intermittent fasting has many significant and positive consequences for your health. People who have it as part of their routine say their minds feel clearer, and they are capable of more productive work because their bodies have more energy. They report an increase in muscle and a decrease in body fat. Insulin goes down, your skin gets shinier and more elastic, and your heart is healthier. And all these benefits came from, when you really break it down, simply skipping a meal or two a day.

We just summarized many of these positive health effects in the previous chapter, but in Chapter 3, we have the opportunity to provide you with even more knowledge about how it will improve your body's health.

Autophagy: Nature's Detoxifier

Now that you have learned the science underlying the benefits of autophagy, we can dive deeper into the cleansing side of it. The science behind it is what makes intermittent fasting better than other strategies to increase your health that end up doing more harm than good. It tells us that it is something that all of us should be thinking about — even if we are not trying to lose weight — because it just has that much influence on our bodies.

Even as you read into the third chapter, I can guarantee you that you have not yet scratched the surface of what it will do for your body once you find yourself doing it every day. Look at it this way: there is definitely a lot of evidence that kale is a superfood that is very good for you since it is filled with so many vitamins and nutrients that your body needs. That's why everyone says that you should eat it.

Some people take scientific facts, like kale being good for you, and twist them to make it seem like kale is the only food you should be eating. They try to sell you diets based on blending kale and drinking it throughout the day. While it's true that consuming more kale would be good for you, it still doesn't compare to autophagy. That's because while this veg is great, it still doesn't give you everything you need, and more importantly, it isn't literally essential to your body.

On the other hand, autophagy is essential to your body. It happens whether you like it or not, and if you never thought about it in your whole life, it would still happen. If your cells didn't go through it, your cells would die, and you would die along with them. This is what makes detoxifying your body with autophagy different from detoxifying your body with something like kale. We are taking something that your body already does and needs and maximizing it to its greatest potential.

No matter how much energy you feel like you are using at any given time, your cells are always using energy. Unlike you and me, they do not get to sleep and recover from a long day. This is what makes autophagy a central part of a cell's functions: when you fast and your cells' food resources are depleted, they still need energy to keep on going — so they find their energy in the nooks and crannies. Your cells eat their own unused proteins, broken organelles, and their autophagosomes start working extra hard to find the toxins that are in various parts of your system. They are extra motivated to do this when you fast because if they don't, they can't keep doing the things that cells do.

Our cells don't care about their state of cleanliness the way you do. You care about their cleanliness because they work much better when they have cleared out the toxins, and that's where all the positive health effects of autophagy come from. But since your cells don't care themselves, they will let things get very crowded: they will have toxins all over and will simply die off when it becomes so much that they can't work properly.

Of course, they will eventually go through some maintenance mode autophagy when you go to sleep. But you are reading this book because you want your cells to go above and beyond what they would do normally — because that is what is going to get the best health outcomes for you.

We really let our cells make a mess of themselves in the modern-day. Once you do your first intermittent fast, you will realize how much we eat every day like it's nothing. To briefly look at things from a philosophical standpoint, we are always filling ourselves with stuff, and we don't give ourselves a chance to empty ourselves out. Autophagy comes in for that last part. Our bodies are not anywhere equipped to deal with all the junk we stuff into our bodies these days, so we have to think about our cells proactively and make sure they use this process to keep things running efficiently.

We all know the artificial chemicals that inevitably end up in our bodies in today's society. If we don't deliberatively take care of it by doing intermittent fasting, some of these may end up having negative long-term consequences on our health. I don't advocate for being paranoid about what chemicals are in our foods, but it is a simple fact that our foods are filled with them, and we can't be certain that all of them are fine for us. It may not be possible for us to get rid of these chemicals in our lives completely, but we can get rid of the ones that do end up in our bodies using the natural cleansing process of autophagy.

Not only will you get rid of these toxins for the sake of your general health, but having a clean system leaves you feeling great, too. You can really feel the difference subjectively. We talk so much about the physical health side of things in this book, but we can't ignore the emotional element. Having the peace of mind that your body is consistently getting rid of toxins can be relieving in trying times. Using IF is not only about optimizing your physical health as much as possible, but your psychological health as well.

When the detox is a big part of what you want autophagy to do for you, you may be motivated to make it as potent as possible by using a variety of triggering methods. IF should be your main method of triggering autophagy since it is the easiest, and therefore, the most reliable. But once you start feeling the difference in your skin and under it — once the work your cells are doing is a sensation you detect throughout your biological systems

— there is a good chance you will fall in love with it and want more.

You can combine intermittent fasting with other techniques to make your detox as powerful as possible. If you have a sauna in your community that you can visit, it could be helpful. Saunas do so much good for your body, as they will make your heart rate go down, improve the circulation of your blood, and do a detox on your body directly through your skin. Saunas do this because they put your cells into a state of stress. If you recall, this state of stress is the thing that puts your cells into autophagy. Intermittent fasting is the best way to trigger the state of stress on a daily, reliable basis, but saunas will help, too, giving you the best natural detox possible.

Even if you don't have a sauna, you can get some of the benefits of taking a hot shower, as the steam will seep into your skin and do some of the detoxification that a sauna would do. Thus, your cells will get some of the state of stress that would come from a sauna. None of this is to say that a sauna or hot shower should replace intermittent fasting — they shouldn't, because they don't advance autophagy as much as fasting. However, if you use these methods alongside intermittent fasting, the autophagy you get will increase.

Autophagy and Your Skin

Now that you know more about the science of it, we can go deeper into the health benefits that IF will confer to your skin.

First of all, you should know how important hydration is to your skin. You may be going through autophagy 12 hours a day and still not see improvement in your skin. Most people do not get enough water every day. Be sure you are drinking 7 glasses a day, at the very least. This is truthfully the best thing you can do for your skin.

Earlier, you learned how the two mechanisms detoxify your system. Well, this means that your pores are cleared out, too. No one wants to keep their pores clogged, and if you drink plenty of water and keep up your habit of intermittent fasting, you won't have to worry about clogged pores in your skin for much longer.

The way that IF improves your skin works in two ways. For one, it unclogs these pores, since autophagy breaks down the toxins that clog them up. But it also makes your skin cells healthier overall. This results in the long-term and more desired effect of more elastic and more youthful skin.

When you keep your skin healthy with autophagy, your true goal is to increase the amount of collagen that your skin cells produce. We went into this topic in the last chapter, but now we have the space to go into more detail.

It is actually not all of your skin cells that produce the collagen protein, but just some of them. These skin cells are called fibroblasts. Fibroblasts are specialized cells made to produce the protein we have been talking about known as collagen.

You can't go wrong with collagen — the more you have of it, the healthier and more elastic your skin is. Even when we turn 18, our fibroblasts start producing less collagen, and our skin starts getting less stretchy as a result. If you want more collagen, you have to take care of your cells by drinking lots of water and doing IF to trigger autophagy. Our fibroblasts stop making as much collagen because they get clogged up with toxins, just like our pores. These cells are not as efficient since they are so crowded out by toxins. The unused proteins, organelles, and other toxins start to add up and create real problems for your fibroblast's functioning.

This is what we mean when we say that autophagy helps your skin in two ways, because one triggers the other to clean out your pores, but this reduction in toxins also ends up making your fibroblasts healthier and more efficient. More efficient cells are able to do their job properly; fibroblasts get better at producing collagen, and your skin gets tighter.

Taking care of your skin is not only a matter of appearance, although there is nothing wrong with wanting to manage your looks too. Your skin is one of your most important organs. Healthier skin protects you against skin cancer, ultraviolet rays, and diseases trying to permeate through your skin cells' membranes.

The cells of your skin organ are a great example in general because skin cells get replaced a lot — all of them get replaced every month. Autophagy is integral to this non-stop process of renewal in your skin cells. Triggering it with IF will result in these health benefits because you are protecting the continuous cycle of skin cells that you need to protect your body.

When you want to detoxify your body, your skin is the best place to do it. It serves as your first line of defense against the toxins that enter your body from the outside.

It is also the best way to get better, healthier skin because it has the capacity to tackle this continual cycle of new cells in your skin. No other method can deal with the constant stream of new skin cells, which is why they tend to fail.

For instance, there are endless skincare products that claim to do what autophagy really does for your skin, but this is impossible since these products can't compete with the way it goes deep into your layers of skin, to your old cells and new cells.

These skincare products can only put creme on top of your outermost layer of skin, making it look better, but it is only covering it up without solving the problem that can only be solved through cellular means.

It is unfortunate that so many people waste their time and money on products that don't work, but at least you won't have to. In fact, the improved health and youthfulness of your skin will probably be the first thing you notice as a result of intermittent fasting. Along with weight loss, it is commonly reported as the first noticeable difference.

The desire to lose weight and get better skin often go together. One reason for this is fear of the so-called "skin curtain." We already discussed this fear briefly, but I want to be sure that you do not let this irrational fear hold you back from making lifestyle changes that are good for your body. Like we said before, loose skin from weight loss has a lot of factors that go into it: (1) the speed at which you lose the weight, (2) how much weight is lost, (3) genetics, (4) age, and (5) the health of your skin. Not only can we deal with loose skin to once you have it, a lot of these things can be prevented in the first place. We can control them. Let's get into controlling loose skin once we have it, though.

Probably the biggest reason we shouldn't worry about loose skin from weight loss is that it isn't permanent. Of course, these things always go on a case-by-case basis, but most people who are looking at loose skin after weight loss don't have to accept it into their lives. There are a variety of ways that it can be managed once you have it, and surgery isn't the only option. Working to do without of loose skin is a lot like taking care of your skin in general. You want to drive 7 or more glasses of water a day, be getting exercise, get the essential nutrients you should be getting anyway.

It takes time to tighten up your loose skin, for sure, but this is a much easier problem to deal with than excess fat on your body. It is incredible how many people are reluctant to slim down because of their irrational fear of loose skin; don't let yourself be one of them. In short, loose skin can be handled once you lose the weight. It is not permanent, just like being overweight or obese isn't permanent. Just like those things, you just have to put in the work consistently and be patient as time does its part in tightening up loose skin from weight loss.

You can keep the loose skin from being a problem in the first place, too. Your age and how much weight you need to lose are not things that you can control, but you can control other things: how much water you drink, how quickly you lose the weight, whether you get enough nutrients, and whether you exercise.

Most importantly, you can do the first method trigger the other, and this will help with loose skin the most. It has been shown in research that people who fast deal with less loose skin when they lose the weight they want to lose. Take care of the things you can control, and if you still have some loose skin when the weight is off, keep taking care of your body and following your IF routine so your skin tightens as quickly as possible.

You can pay attention to how you feel when you fast to help prevent loose skin in the first place. Many people say that when they do a longer fast like a water fast that their skin feels strange. You can feel this slightly without worrying about it, but if the feeling goes further than that, you might want to stop your fast early. It could be that your skin is not adjusting to your new body shape quickly enough, and if the fast continues, you will have the loose skin that you don't want.

It's true that your skin is the organ that everyone can see, and this is why there is a multi-million-dollar industry to help people improve their skin health. However, the way your skin looks should not be the main thing that you are concerned about. It is just like how people want to lose weight to look better but losing weight will also decrease their health risks for heart disease and cancer, too. Women, in particular, need to pay close attention to the health of their skin, because sometimes they use so many products on them that they are unsure of the natural state of their skin health.

After you take a shower, inspect your skin and evaluate how healthy you think it is. Inspecting your skin regularly will get you motivated to keep on your IF regimen. You will see improvements very quickly. Your skin's purpose is not to look nice, but to protect your body from toxins on the outside. Doing IF will help you protect your skin, empowering it to shield your system from pathogens and microbes. Thankfully, taking care of your skin will also make it look better. It is a win-win situation.

Autophagy and Your Energy

Everyone who fasts says the same thing: they can do so much more now every day than they used to be able to because they have more energy.

You already know that everything that you do requires energy — and this is true all the way down to your cells. Your cells, in a sense, need more energy than you do, because they have to keep doing their jobs 24/7. They will break down organelles and proteins that no longer help them when you deprive them of food because they always need to find energy somewhere.

If you don't generate autophagy except when you are sleeping, a lot of negative consequences are likely — one of them being low energy. Many people who don't have much energy feel this way because their cells are not running optimally. Their cells are having to drag along all their cellular waste getting in the way. If you don't fast to force them to clean this out, they will still do it, but not nearly enough.

The mitochondria are where all of your energy starts. This is the organelle where your cell makes energy so it can perform all the jobs that it has to do. This chapter focuses on the benefits for your body, but it is useful to think about things from a microscopic point of view, too. The mitochondrion is arguably the most important organelle in your cells. If your mitochondrion is working well, this is a sign that your cell is working well. When scientists look at mitochondrial health in people, they find that those with well-functioning mitochondria are at low risk for neurodegenerative diseases like Huntington's, Alzheimer's, and Parkinson's.

Your mitochondria do their job best when they don't have to deal with clutter. Clutter builds up around your mitochondria in their cell from all the sources we have mentioned, and this slows it down. When you don't generate autophagy enough, this has consequences for mitochondria all over your body — consequences for the one place where all your energy ultimately comes from. It's no wonder that people who fast have more energy. Their cells' power plants are working better than they ever have before!

It is likely that you have heard of ATP before. ATP is the particle that is fundamental to your body's energy at an atomic level. ATP is where all of your cells get their energy. It doesn't matter whether your cells get energy from breaking down your food or from breaking down toxins — ATP is at the center of the process.

The details of ATP breakdown are truly fascinating, but for our purposes, we can summarize by saying that your cells use the energy that comes from converting ATP into ADP and back into ATP again (and so on).Now, this process of ATP breakdown doesn't require energy because it's how we get energy, but it does require two things: oxygen and nourishment. All living things break down ATP, be they animals or plants. The main difference is animals use oxidation, and plants use photosynthesis.

The fascinating truth about ATP is that your system generates around 170 pounds of it each day, despite the fact that there are only around 9 ounces of ATP in your body at any given time. You only ever have half a pound of ATP in your body, yet the process of transformation of ATP, giving your body energy goes through the weight of a human. The process of ATP breakdown occurs in the mitochondria of all of your cells. When you let ATP happen using toxins, dead organelles, and proteins during intermittent fasting, this makes the process much more effective.

Remember: your cells don't have brains like you do, because if they did, they would know that they should clean themselves out to make ATP breakdown happen more smoothly. But now that you know this yourself, this is no longer a problem. Make IF a regular part of your life and start seeing your energy levels spike.

Autophagy: It's What's Good for You

The fact is, not everyone thinks as much about their general health as they should. The sad thing is that once you are diagnosed with something that could have been prevented, you wish that you had thought more about taking care of your body.

If you are reading now and you aren't currently looking at a major health crisis, the good thing is that it isn't too late yet, as you can still turn around your attitude of health and start caring about it. We are primarily focused on what autophagy can do for your health through intermittent fasting, but the habits that make it more potent are the same ones that you should keep up for the betterment of your health in general.

It should be enough to tell you that intermittent fasting reduces your risk for neurodegenerative diseases. The older you get, the higher your chances of getting one of these becomes. It is within your power to lower your risk, and these new habits don't just increase the length of your life. They make you feel better too, improving the quality of your life.

We won't spend too much more time on Alzheimer's and the rest since we have already talked about them a lot, but diabetes is a disease that should not be taken lightly, either. Many people live with diabetes, but that doesn't mean it has no consequences. If you don't have it already, it is certainly worth the change in lifestyle to avoid it.

IF is a great path to staying away from diabetes. People who get this disease end up with amyloid deposits in their arteries, but if their cells had broken down the amyloid during autophagy, they wouldn't have gotten diabetes in the first place. Scientists are still learning more about the potential of this process to treat these diseases, but what we can already do is stop them in their tracks through fasting.

You can look at the positive effects of it on your overall health from two different angles. First and most obviously, there is the angle of stopping microbes and pathogens before they become an issue. If your body is in the mode of autophagy half the time because you are passionate about it and fasting, there is a very good chance you will rarely have to worry about infection — because your cells always deal with them very early.

This is the purpose of the advanced one. So, you will go through what biologists call "maintenance mode" autophagy no matter what your body habits are. No one in the world eats every moment of the day, and everyone has to sleep. During these periods of time, our cells still need energy, so they have to go through it to get food with which to go through ATP breakdown.

Intermittent fasting spurs the biological process that puts a stopper on many risks for age-related disease: high inflammation, high blood pressure, being overweight, and more. Autophagy's lowering of inflammation is often underappreciated in research. Inflammation is something that can speed up the progression of disease when something else is wrong. You may have an infection, but if you have a relatively low level of inflammation, there is a good chance that your body will eventually take care of it. If you have high inflammation and you get an infection, however, the issue is compounded. Your system is sluggish and doesn't fight off the pathogen before it is too late.

The earlier you start IF, the better, because your autophagy won't be as potent at first. Even if you do everything right — paying attention to your nutrients, not consuming too many calories, exercising, drinking enough water, and following your IF regimen — your first month or so of fasting won't do nearly as much as the months after. It takes time for your body to break toxins down. If you had not ever fasted before, your autophagy is now working on a backlog of old toxins that will take time to get there. Luckily, once this is finished, it will be better than ever.

And on the subject of inflammation, once autophagy decreases your inflammation, it will be more effective as well. If you have not talked to your doctor about inflammation before, you might not be sure if yours is high or not. You might have high inflammation if you have bad habits like smoking, overeating, alcohol abuse, or following a sedentary lifestyle.

Some of the most recent studies about this system have shown that a low amount of it is the cause of neurodegenerative diseases. I may have already made clear that it fights against these diseases, but now you should know precisely why. It all has to do with a special kind of it: chaperone-mediated autophagy. We will go into more detail on what this distinction means later one. This is what you need to know for now, though — biologists found that the gene instructing your cells to go through chaperone-mediated autophagy was damaged in people with neurodegenerative diseases. Since the gene was damaged, they did not go through the chaperone-mediated one when they should have. Next, proteins piled up inside the brain cells of people with these diseases. The buildup of protein gets to a point where the brain cells don't work properly anymore, and they die.

There is another theory on how it happens, but it has the same result. Other scientists think that the autophagosome (transporter essential to chaperone-mediated autophagy and macro-autophagy) binds to the lysosome (cell stomach) too strongly. As a result, there is a clogging effect, and too many proteins crowded into a cell, leading to its dysfunction and eventual death. It can be tempting to think that such things are inevitable. It can seem like you can't do anything about what happens in your brain cells. You think, just let it be. It is outside of my control. But this is not true at all. There are many people who do not ever get these diseases. Of course, we cannot deny that genes play a role, but saying that genes determine everything is just a way of not doing what we can.

Let's assume that the scientists who say neurodegeneration happens because of the "clogging effect" are right. The way you should look at it is that you can still prevent the issue from getting out of hand, just like you can with infections. When the clogging effect happens in people's brain cells, it doesn't happen in every single one.

This gives you the opportunity to generate autophagy in the cells without the clogging effect so they can clean out the protein buildups before they get out of hand. If you do this on a regular basis, you won't have to have the stress of a damaged gene.

Your cells inevitably age just like we do and get damaged genes. This doesn't mean that we should give up on them and simply allow them to not work as well as they could. Our cells without damaged DNA can pick up the slack for the ones who do. Besides, the chaperone-mediated one has another role that we have not yet gotten to. Scientists were excited to see that this special kind of process is actually responsible for repairing your cells' DNA.

If you use IF regularly — especially if you are making autophagy unleash to its fullest extent — you can even repair the genes that prevent it from working the way it should. The two methods can teach all of us to take more initiative with our health. When you learn how much control we really have, it can serve as quite a wake-up call. All you need is the knowledge of how it works and the will to live healthily for as long as possible.

Chapter 4

Intermittent Fasting and Autophagy

At the heart of intermittent fasting's benefits is the science that makes all of it work. Autophagy is the biological process in which your cells, when unable to get energy from food, consume "junk" materials such as unused organelles, proteins, and foreign toxins.

You put your body through this biological process when you do intermittent fasting because you are depriving your cells of food to consume, so they switch to autophagy to get their energy. Because of this, you can reap all the advantages of it by simply not eating during certain windows of the day.

This will be the chapter where we dive into the biological component of intermittent fasting, the process that we aim to achieve by fasting autophagy. I know that science is not everyone's cup of tea, but you need to know this essential information, so you know how to best set up your IF routine.

Even if you are a fan of learning about science, it is easy to get overwhelmed with information overload, but there are some simple facts that will make things easier for you. Firstly, I am not leaving out anything important in this chapter, you can rest easy knowing that you are not missing something important about autophagy in this chapter.

The other simple fact is that I am still only telling you what you need to know. Put together, what I'm saying is that you don't need to check other sources to learn the science of autophagy, because this one is exhaustive, and you don't need to worry about reading more information than you can absorb, because I am telling you what you need to know and nothing more. This science-based chapter is woven in such a way that you do not have to worry about accidentally skipping something important. Everything is connected and related to each other. So, all you have to do is continue reading the chapter from start to finish, and your job is done.

Part of the reason learning the science behind intermittent fasting is so important is because you need to be certain of autophagy's significance yourself. If you can't tell your friends in a few sentences why you are doing IF, you will lose sight of the purpose of it, and you might be in danger of stopping. You will have more than a few sentences to say to back up this science after reading this chapter. It is probable that you might annoy your friends with facts about autophagy for a week or so after reading.

They might be annoyed with you, but they won't be able to discredit the points your making, so you will probably be doing their health a favor. Doing IF is a lot more fun when you have friends or family doing it with you, so learning the ins and outs of the science behind it is a great opportunity to recruit others to help you live more healthily.

Where It All Started

There is a history that accompanies the study of autophagy and all the things we know about it regarding our health. It was a term that people might use for its philosophical meaning that can be gleaned from "self" "eat" (autophagy), but even using the term to refer to a specific biological phenomenon is a new thing.

The first scientist to get close to learning about this process is Christian De Duve, and he was the first one to use this term. However, his understanding of it is so different from what we think of it now, that it is almost like he was studying something else entirely. In France in the 1960's, Christian De Duve saw a new organelle while looking at yeast cells in the laboratory. Since it had never been identified before, his team of researchers started learning all the bizarre things about it. They called this organelle the "lysosome." The lysosome was understood quite differently back then, though. Christian De Duve still called the lysosome the center of autophagy because he concluded that this was the garbage receptacle of the cell.

You can see how scientists got some things right, but most things wrong. It makes sense, given that they had only just discovered the site of it, but biological understanding has gone far past seeing the lysosome and autophagy this way.

It was very recently that our understanding evolved to what it is today. The Japanese scientists Yoshinori Ohsumi won the Nobel Prize for re-defining autophagy into how we see it today. Ohsumi studied yeast cells too, but unlike Christian De Duve, yeast cells were the basis of his entire career. To this day, his team is still trying to learn more about it, and they are still using yeast cells to do this. From reading so far, you already know what Ohsumi learned from looking at the lysosomes of yeast cells. We now know that it is not simply a process of disposal, but a process of recycling.

This makes a lot more sense, too, because there is no such thing as "breaking something down" in the real world so it turns into nothing. We can only change the form of matter; we can't actually destroy it. Ohsumi incorporated the "recycling" aspect of autophagy by being the first to talk about what he calls the "cell cycle." The cell cycle is the means by which your cells break down their toxins in the lysosome and then use the raw materials left behind to build new things. With the raw materials collected from it, our cells can build new organelles and new cells.

The cell cycle is how our cells use their waste to create cellular structures, and then those structures break down their waste to create their own structures, and so forth. It is interesting that we did not think of our cells this way until the last few years, because in retrospect, we know that it is one of the essential jobs that your cells must do.

Ohsumi's research has gotten pharmacists started on medicines that can use our knowledge of autophagy to fight aging and age-related disease. They could find something revolutionary that could change medicine forever any day. In the meantime, we can make the best use out of what we already know.

Now that you know the context under which it has been studied — and now that you know how cutting-edge autophagy really is — we will explore the different kinds of it that exist and how they apply to IF.

Micro-autophagy

This is the form that autophagy takes in every single cell of your body. All cells have lysosomes, and those lysosomes have the chief purpose of conducting micro-autophagy. As usual, their job is to bring in damaged organelles to break them down. This is different from macro-autophagy and chaperone-mediated autophagy, where the lysosome does not pull in the cellular waste on its own. In those kinds of autophagy, a special organelle called the autophagosome has the job of finding waste inside and outside of the cell. Then, it carries them over to the lysosome and binds with it to break down its contents.

This form happens in every cell because it does some very important jobs. It helps with the homeostasis of the membrane and it keeps the cell's organelles at their current size.

The chemical function of the lysosome is still being studied, but essentially its method of breaking down the cellular waste is attacking them with enzymes. Finally, micro-autophagy is finished and the cell uses the raw materials attained from breaking down the waste for its part of the cell cycle. The cell can use the materials for building a new cell, building a new organelle, or for building even more basic things like glucose, amino acids, fatty acids, and so forth.

Macro-autophagy

Macro-autophagy is the type of autophagy that is only seen in cells with certain jobs. This type and chaperone-mediated autophagy use the autophagosome. The autophagosome can be simply described as a vesicle — that is, it can carry things inside of it and transport them. This vesicle (the autophagosome) travels around inside the cell and goes outside the cell to find waste to break down when you are fasting, and food is scarce. When it is done wandering through the cytoplasm finding waste, it returns to the lysosome and binds with it.

When the autophagosome takes the materials into the lysosome, this is called sequestration; it has a double membrane around it that it uses to trap materials inside. When sequestration occurs, both membranes open so that the lysosome can take the toxins that the vesicle found. But in macro-autophagy, it is not the lysosome that breaks down the toxins, but the autophagosome. It can only break them down when it is bonded to the lysosome, however.

Since it only happens in specialized cells like white blood cells, there are actually a few different kinds of macro-autophagy itself, such as mitophagy and ribophagy. Most of the time, these different kinds of macro-autophagy are made for getting rid of specific organelles that have stopped working.

Chaperone-Mediated Autophagy

The direction of biology and medicine may hinge on our newest findings about this kind of autophagy: chaperone-mediated autophagy. Scientists have known about the other two types of it for much longer than chaperone-mediated autophagy; it was Yoshinori Ohsumi's research that led to the interest in it that spurred its discovery. The findings that we have so far will influence science and medicine for decades to come.

The chaperone-mediated one is the most specialized of the three. Essentially, this kind of autophagy differentiates itself because it uses chains of proteins to move materials into the lysosome. The proteins themselves are specialized for this one purpose in chaperone-mediated autophagy, and the materials they help move into the lysosome are specific proteins that CMA seeks after.

In our chapter about the benefits, we went into CMA briefly because of its job of DNA repair. I am about to go into all the wonders of chaperone-mediated autophagy and what we know about it so far, but we can summarize the most important facts about CMA briefly.

For one, it does not only break down proteins. It has a vital role in repairing DNA. As we learned earlier, the DNA repair of cells is very important, because damaged DNA leads to cells not performing as they should be. When your brain cells have damaged genes, they don't perform autophagy when they should, and the result is buildups of proteins that lead to Alzheimer's, Parkinson's, and Huntington's.

Next, CMA is important because it seeks after specific proteins to break them down. This is crucial because if CMA did not do this, the raw materials from those proteins could be lacking in a cell and it wouldn't be able to proceed in the cell cycle as efficiently.

Besides these two important jobs, chaperone-mediated autophagy has some others, too. Studies have concluded that CMA plays a role in your cell metabolism and in controlling your glucose levels. Keeping your glucose relatively low is what makes autophagy possible in the first place.

Micro-autophagy and macro-autophagy might end up breaking down important proteins for the raw materials they need, but they can't use specialized protein chains to seek specific proteins out.

Cells that perform CMA know which proteins to seek out because of the instructions from their genes. It is useful that CMA is also needed to repair the DNA of cells, because it needs that DNA to do its job.

In the last chapter, we learned that the precursor to Alzheimer's and similar diseases is damaged DNA inside cells. I told you that you shouldn't accept this as something you can't control, because using autophagy, you do have the power to fight against damaged DNA and eventual neurodegeneration.

You can use this book as a life-changing resource to optimize the effects of it and repair your cell DNA as often as possible. Anything you could ever need to know about how to do this is contained in here.

While we are getting more in the weeds about the chaperone-mediated process, you should learn about the latest gene related to it: LAMP-2A. This name stands for lysosome-associated membrane protein.

We know a few things about this gene already: (1) it has a strong link to chaperone-mediated autophagy and (2) when scientists preserve this gene in lab mice, they had better outcomes in health and longer lifespans than mice without having this gene protected. One scientist even noted that the mice whose LAMP-2A was protected had "healthier-looking fur" and "a glow about them."

If these symptoms sound familiar, it's because they are close to the ones that humans experience when they trigger autophagy by fasting. Your skin gets a glow, and while we don't have fur, there's a good chance the new hair you grow will be healthier, too.

When I told you that chaperone-mediated autophagy could repair DNA, regulate metabolism, and control glucose levels, all of these jobs are actually due to instructions that your cells get from their LAMP-2A gene. It's also the gene that probably gets damaged in people who develop neurodegenerative diseases.

The LAMP-2A gene is supposed to tell your specialized cells to start chaperone-mediated autophagy and seek out the specific proteins named in their DNA. When these genes are damaged, your autophagy does not function as it is supposed to, and all the biological processes that rely on it start to have problems as well.

Some of the recent findings have turned out to be incredibly relevant to matters of personal health. It has only been in the past decade that we found out that Alzheimer's and Parkinson's disease are a result of a mutation in a gene that controls autophagy.

Let's step back for a second and define what we mean by mutation. As we age, the DNA in our cells becomes damaged from wear and tear. One of the genes in our DNA is the one that controls autophagy. When that gene takes damage, our autophagy is less effective because it is not getting proper instructions from the DNA.

As a result, when your brain cells create protein chains to do certain jobs, these protein chains become clusters that are toxic to your cells, all because these cells did not have undamaged genes from which to take their instructions.

Now you might worry that this gene damage as a result of age means that there is nothing you can do about it, but this could not be further from the truth. Your takeaway from this scientific discovery should be that you need to manually turn on autophagy as you get older because your cells' genes will not be as effective at doing it automatically. You can turn on it through fasting and exercise and get the same much-needed autophagy as you would if your genes instructed your cells to do it to themselves.

Microscopic is Everything

Perhaps you are a reader who is skeptical about something so small having such an impact. You believe that all the science is true, but you don't think that your cells are what you should focus on, when you could focus on your specific organs or certain muscles.

It might help for you to think of yourself as one big cell. As you, the cell, age, you take damage. Cells that have gone through damage do not work as well until they go through autophagy and fix their injuries.

In much the same way, you as a person can suffer injuries, and those injuries impede your ability to do what you need to do. If you got in an accident tomorrow and broke your hand, there are a lot of things you wouldn't be able to do, even if you don't have to go to work, things that used to be simple — like getting the mail — are not simple anymore.

A cell with an injury to the mitochondria is not in the right state to cooperate with the rest of your cells. Ultimately, we are talking about just one cell here, and it doesn't do any good alone — especially if it is injured and not working properly.

It might seem like one cell doesn't matter, but you have over 30 trillion cells in your whole body. That's 30,000,000,000,000 cells.

You aren't made of anything else, either. Just cells. Even though one cell admittedly doesn't matter, issues arise when cells throughout your body aren't getting enough autophagy.

There is even a process of programmed cell death that your cell might run if they are too damaged to help the rest of the tissue. They also might do this if they are starting to become a cancer cell; that way, they do not hurt the rest of the body.

Since autophagy disposes of cellular waste and builds new cell structures throughout all of your cells, it is your best defense against threats to your health: and it happens in your microscopic cells. There is no real way to talk about your autophagy outside of your cells, at least when it comes to biology.

You can't do a single thing you do without your cells, so don't underestimate them. Don't underestimate the harmful effects of DNA damage in your cells and the buildup of toxins inside them.

When we age, our cells get less effective. Consequently, they are less effective because their organelles are so. When you have a mitochondrion or another organelle that does not perform well, it is really better to break it down and make it a new mitochondrion. Getting your cells to do this will result in better overall health for you.

However, your cells don't know this like you do. If you want them to dispose of the bad orangeades that are making them lag behind, you have to trigger autophagy by yourself. You have already learned some of the methods that people can use to do this: intermittent fasting, water fasting, a nutrient-rich diet, exercise, a hot shower, or even a sauna will do the trick.

Your cells might not take care of their poorly performing organelles if you do not use these techniques. They might continue using the same old mitochondria without even improving it. When a lot of your cells do this, you end up feeling a difference subjectively.

The health of your cells is the health of your body. You can't micromanage trillions of cells, but you can be a puppet master and manipulate them to do what you want as best as you can.

Take a broken-down vehicle as an example. You might feel emotionally attached to a car that stopped working, but that doesn't mean that you should hold onto it forever. For the first few times that it broke down, you bought the new parts and simply fixed the car. It didn't work as well as before, and it made some suspicious noises, but you like the car, so you allowed it.

But then there is the final straw. You have put thousands of dollars into the car, and at this point, even though you have an attachment to it, you can't justify spending all this money on a car that will just keep breaking down soon after you fix it.

You might say that your cells get attached to their organelles. They don't literally, of course, but they certainly won't get rid of them until they absolutely have to.

This illustrates your cells working in maintenance mode. When you use all of the methods to trigger advanced autophagy together, you can basically communicate with your cells, saying: "I want you to take out the trash."

Your cells need the energy, and they will dig into their reserves. If you spent many years without fasting and without following a generally healthy lifestyle, there is a good chance that it will take time for your cells to break down their problematic organelles. That's because they have so many other options for energy that have stacked up over the years.

After you do intermittent fasting for enough time, though, your cells will finally run out of options and break down their mitochondria. Then, they will use the parts to build a new one. You will surely feel a difference after just a week or so doing IF, but this is why the biggest difference in energy levels will be after a longer period of time.

You have likely heard before that humans can live for three weeks or so without eating anything. Autophagy is the reason this is true. At the end of the day, it isn't "you" who has to eat, but your cells, as they keep your body alive for weeks because there is plenty already inside of you that they can consume for energy.

But it isn't only when you are starving that your cells break down this much material. Did you know that we need around 100 grams of protein each day? It sounds like a lot, but the reason the number is so high is that you actually only get about one-third of this protein from the foods that you consume.

The only two-thirds of the proteins that your body breaks down every day are protein already inside you. This is autophagy. Even before you knew what it was, it was supplying twice the volume of protein than you were consuming yourself. In other words, your cells don't just break down the protein you eat once. They break it down several times until it is eventually converted into a useful structure, then that cellular structure stops functioning in the required way, autophagy breaks it down, and it continues on and on.

Another strange thing about this microscopic phenomenon is that you don't have to do anything special to get your body to do it. It is doing it right now, and it will continue to do it for as long as you live. You didn't do anything special to harm your proteins and organelles, either — they simply accrued damage over time while you were going about your normal life.

This phenomenon is an essential biological process that will continue whether you decide to pay attention to it or not. But think about this: why would you not want to pay close attention to a process this important? A process that has been instrumental in keeping you alive to this point?

You have the option to add to the power of it by changing your way of living, such as your eating habits and your exercise habits. We all know that the older we get, the more work we have to do to make our bodies perform the way that they should. But usually, we hear this about our organs, our bones, and our muscles. For some reason, no one says this about autophagy — even though none of these systems would function without it.

The Newest Science

It can be exciting to learn about new scientific discoveries, and the newer the discoveries are, the more exciting they are. This is our final section in the chapter about the science underlying the IF, and it will concentrate on the newest information that we have about autophagy.

Just keep in mind that these findings are the definition of cutting-edge, meaning there is probably more information about them by the time you read this. You might want to do some research for yourself to see if anything new has been discovered. With that said, at the time of writing, these are the latest findings we have.

To begin, there is another important gene in autophagy besides the LAMP-2A gene. It is called ATG. ATG doesn't stand for anything — it's just supposed to look like the word "autophagy" since its main purpose is to instruct it.

The ATG gene is often discussed alongside the protein chain VPS-34. Both of them are needed to provoke it and keep it regulated. While scientists protected the LAMP-2A gene from improving the overall health of mice, they found that they could get the most out of VPS-34 by

202

altering it. The manipulation of this protein chain may be key to treating or even curing age-related diseases.

VPS-34 is an easily manipulated chain, and this makes it a great tool for biologists trying to learn more about this process. We know that the beginning of many of the diseases we are talking about is related to the deterioration of functions related to chaperone-mediated autophagy. The ability to manipulate one of the protein chains related to CMA (VPS-34) is a phenomenal step in the right direction for everyone who wants to end diseases like cancer.

Some say that it is only a matter of time before experiments on VPS-34 lead to a new ground-breaking discovery. When that happens, medicine as we know it — especially as it relates to aging — will be totally changed.

There is one more gene you should know: the P62 gene. This gene is often attributed to the relatively long lifespan that humans have compared to other mammals.

It took time for humans to get the P62 gene in our evolution, but what does it do? Maybe you won't be surprised that it is related to chaperone-mediated autophagy: it lets our cells know when there are dangerous products that could harm them, causing them to go into a state of stress and trigger autophagy.

When scientists created genetically mutated fruit flies and gave them the P62 gene, they survived for longer than fruit flies without the P62 gene. This experiment alone should convince you of the singular potential of the well-known phenomenon.

Now that you have a strong grasp on the research for cancer and neurodegenerative diseases, we should spend some time on another important disease: diabetes. Then, I will recommend what foods to eat when you are following a routine of intermittent fasting in the next chapter.

You might remember learning about amyloid deposits, the buildups of proteins that lead to diabetes. There is a lesson to be learned in all these cases of diseases that could be prevented with more autophagy; they are not caused by a foreign invader. They are caused by our bodies working seemingly normally — until an invisible line is crossed, and too much protein accumulates in the cells.

If there is only one takeaway you have from this science-focused chapter, it should be that increased autophagy prevents the diseases that we can't otherwise address until it's too late.

You can't tell when your proteins are crowded out your brain cells or cells anywhere else; the only way you can prevent it from becoming a problem is by fasting regularly. If you do that, you will know that you are doing everything you can do to stave off diseases for which there is no other real treatment.

Chapter 5

Food to Eat During Intermittent Fasting

If there is one thing to remember in an intermittent fast, it's this: lower your consumption of carbohydrates. The reason for this is that carbs take a long time for your body to process, and as long as your body is processing food, it is not starting autophagy yet.

This ends up reducing the amount of time your body goes through it. Carbs are also the first thing your gut decides to break down — it will break down carbs before protein or fat. With that important tip in mind, let's get into the best foods to eat if you want to maximize the good your body gets from intermittent fasting.

Your general guiding principle needs to be that you have to stop eating without thinking — that is, you need to recognize the different physical and mental consequences that you will have because of the foods that you eat. Once you get really good at following this principle, all the other tips that you hear just seem like common sense.

To quickly review the food we previously told you help with autophagy, they are the reishi mushroom, turmeric, green tea, caffeine, olive oil, and ginger.

All of these foods contain chemicals that will help your body have better autophagy when you trigger it, but they will not do it alone — not without fasting or exercise. Don't get that mixed up.

There are still more foods that you might consider. Grapes have also been found to help, for example. CBD, the non-psychoactive brother of THC, is proved to benefit as well. CBD works particularly well for this purpose because it lessens the amount of inflammation in your body while also improving your neural connections leading the charge to autophagy.

You don't want to spend too much time thinking about what special foods to eat — at least not until you get to a point with IF where you can trust yourself to do it without slipping. When that happens, it can be an exciting way to mix things up.

Ultimately, eating these foods is just doing extra to make your autophagy more advanced. More important than eating these specific foods is getting a balanced diet when you are not inside your fasting window. The rest of the chapter will focus on this because it is much more important.

The best diet for intermittent fasting isn't just the best diet because it is a diet filled with the foods that you should be getting, whether you fast or not.

To get the full potential of autophagy while you do IF, you are best off following this plan, but it does not have to constrain you absolutely. As we said before, the choices you make with your body are yours to make. Even saying that, though, there are certain foods you want to make sure not to eat because they will interfere badly.

I won't make too fine a point on carbs, because you get the message at this point. There is just one other thing to add, which is that even if you fall out of fasting sometime in the future, you still want to greatly reduce the proportion of it in your diet.

They say that Americans are overweight because of sugar and fats, and this is partly true, but the true culprit is carbohydrates. Carbs are the "fluff" of nutrients — they take up a lot of space compared to others, and it is very easy to get too much of it.

Do not misinterpret this and think that you should stay away from carbs altogether. You need carbs just like you need all of these foods. However, it is very easy to get the carbs that you need daily without even trying.

Carbs are a lot like protein this way — it isn't hard to figure out where you will get them, most of the time, because they are in a lot of the foods around us.

It is time for you to learn about protein cycling. Protein cycling is a diet change that many people make when they do IF. Basically, it means alternating between days of normal protein intake and low protein intake.

It is still important that you eat a normal amount of protein on the normal days because protein is an essential nutrient in your body. You need some level of normal protein every day, so your cells have it to build structures.

However, the low-protein days are important too. Having days where you consume little protein will further spur your cells to turn on the process during your fasting window.

Your cells already have plenty of protein lying around as cellular garbage, so your cells can reliably use this as their source of protein on your low-protein days. (Don't forget the fact we learned earlier — your body processes 100 grams of it each day, and only a quarter of that comes from the food you eat!)

With all that in mind, you never want to consume lots of protein, no matter how important a nutrient it is. There is a very good reason for this, as when you eat lots of protein, all you are doing is giving your cells lots of cellular garbage to clean out.

Your cells have to cycle between normal, non-stressed periods and autophagy periods, so it takes time for your cells to dispose of all of this excess.

When they take too long to do it, it eventually becomes toxic, as we have learned. Despite how essential a nutrient protein is, there is such thing as too much of a good thing, especially when it comes to protein.

When your diet is very high in protein, this hampers the progress of autophagy greatly. It does not hamper its progress as much as carbohydrates do, but it still slows things down. Instead of cleaning out your existing cellular garbage when you do IF, you will simply be cleaning out the junk left behind by all the protein you just ate.

Protein cycling gives us a great chance to discuss the importance of finding a balance between IF and a healthy diet. When you do protein cycling, you still need to eat the recommended amount of protein for a reason: it is an essential nutrient.

However, you can go too far in either direction. A lot of the foods people love contain protein, so it is common for people to eat far more protein than they should without even realizing it.

On the other hand, starving yourself of protein to the extreme is harmful, too. If you do this, you may experience loss in muscle tone that is usually associated with fasts more extreme than intermittent fasting.

To do protein cycling right, simply eat the recommended amount of protein every other day, and half or less that amount on your other days.

This is not only about protein, though. Even though IF is a fast meant for everyone, there are still ways we can take it too far. Take someone who makes their fasting window too long: let's say, 14 hours. That would mean they eat for an hour in the morning and then eat again for an hour before bed. This is absolutely unhealthy, and I strongly recommend avoiding it.

I especially advise against it because the IF is meant to be done every day. If you are fasting for 14 hours every day, that could have serious consequences on your body. With a water fast, you may fast for as much as 24 or 48 hours, but the difference is the frequency. Someone can do a water fast all day on Sunday and then go back to their normal eating patterns on Monday.

But if they do IF for 14 hours a day, there is never a time they return to their regular eating pattern. Their regular eating pattern involves consuming far too infrequently.

Maybe you are familiar with the concept of yin and yang from Taoism. The yang gives, and the yin takes. To find a balance between a healthy diet and IF, keep thinking of eating as yang and IF as yin. You need yang to fill yourself up with fresh nutrients.

When you are following it, you do this outside of your fasting window. You need yin to cleanse your cells of the toxins produced from yang.

Too much of yang (eating) and too much of yin (fasting) both have negative consequences. The key is to find a balance between the two; this will allow you to get the benefits of both.

Put another way, don't let yourself believe that "extra" fasting will lead to better health outcomes. It won't. If you truly want to be healthy, you need to find the right about eating for your yang and the right amount of fasting for your yin.

There are writers on the subject of water fasting who concede that these drinks will stymie autophagy to some extent, but they say that at the end of the day, it doesn't make much of a difference. I beg to differ. We have a lot of scientific evidence of the effectiveness of pure water fasting — we don't have any evidence to back up a pure water fast, minus some coffee here and there.

Even a cup of coffee at the beginning of your fast can mess things up. Don't take the risk when you are already looking to get as much as possible out of autophagy.

Another common mistake is consuming flavored water during the water fast. Do not do this — again, the flavoring has something that your body has to break down. When your body breaks down chemicals, autophagy stops. You should even stay away from smells of flavor. It sounds bizarre, but even the smell of real or artificial food causes a parasympathetic reaction from your vagus nerve.

This reaction will actually keep autophagy from happening to a significant degree because it stimulates mTOR, a gene that will stop it when activated. It may feel like there is such a delicate balance, but if you are water fasting to maximize the potential of it, these are the things you have to consider.

Don't even take vitamins or supplements that purport to boost autophagy during your water fast. Not to beat a dead horse, but: your body has to process that, and then it won't start until it's done.

People who advocate for these supplements say that supplements don't have enough digestible chemicals to stop this method from happening, but they don't really know this is the case. They are just selling a supplement. (On a side note, there is no official supplement that is known to turn on or even aid the method at this moment, so you shouldn't bother shopping around for them.)

The list of what to avoid goes on. If it doesn't occur naturally and it comes in colorful packaging, stay away from it. Don't drink soda, eat candy, or buy any of the meat from your grocery store that comes from factory farms. All the nutrients you should be indirectly getting from the grass that animal ate is not there, because these animals are stuffed with chemicals instead of fed grass.

It should probably go without saying, but you need to stay away from sugar as well. Ideally, most of the sugars in your diet come from fruits, and you don't even want to eat too many of those. Even eating more than a little bit of fruit can put too much sugar into your system, so that should tell you how bad sugar is for you.

Sugar may not take as long to digest as carbs, but at least as far as artificial sugars go, you simply don't need it. When you consume too much sugar, you are adding a lot of waste that your cells will have to clean out later.

In fact, this is the image that you should conjure with all of the foods you put into your system. Imagine your broken-down, microscopic foods inside your cells. What will be the most useful to your cells (again, your cells make up all of you): sugary foods or foods with tons of vitamins?

We all know the answer, but the harder part is following through. Actually, doing it may not be as hard as you think. Once you have made the decision to do your first intermittent fasting day tomorrow, you should go grocery shopping. This is what makes it easy: all you have to do is refrain from buying the foods that we are talking about.

Don't buy bagels. Don't buy packaged snacks. Don't buy cake mix.

You know what you should buy already. Put dairy products in your cart that have healthy protein. Put in some natural fruit juice and cucumbers. Pick up healthy nuts like cashews. Find a recipe that you think looks tasty and uses the foods that you want to take part of your normal diet.

Recipes are the key to changing your diet. This is for many reasons. Firstly, cooking takes time, and nothing is better than already knowing how to cook something and already having the ingredients. You will also feel good about making food at home, saving money by not going out.

Going out to eat is a big risk, particularly in the early stages of intermittent fasting. I advise you not to go out to eat until you can at least keep yourself from eating during your fast for two weeks.

Now, let's get right to it. What should you be eating when you do the IF?

I know it's not food, but it deserves as much attention, if not more: water. Every system that keeps you alive needs water to keep going, and that doesn't stop being true when you are fasting. The color of your urine will tell you if you are drinking enough water. The clearer it is, the better — although if it is totally clear, that means you are drinking more than enough water.

Another boon of drinking a lot of water during IF is that it keeps your cravings away. A lot of the times we think that we want food, but what we really feel is thirst.

Next, you need to make fish a weekly dish. They are your best source of Omega-3 fats, an important nutrient for autophagy. Fish also have vitamins and protein. The American Heart Association tells us we should be eating at least one serving of fish every week. Are you?

You may not expect this one, but potatoes are a good food option, too. They are because are especially filling, while actually giving us real nutrients. Getting full on potatoes will keep you from eating when you are supposed to be fasting. There is even research showing that people with potatoes in their diets have more success in losing weight.

We will put legumes and beans in the same category, as most people think of them as the same thing, anyway. Beans are a notably good source of energy while somewhat paradoxically being low in calories. Much like potatoes, beans have been shown to be part of diets where people succeeded in losing weight.

You might already know this, but you still have to be somewhat careful with beans and legumes because they are high in carbs. But I still say they are good for intermittent fasting for all the reasons listed.

Now we are on to nuts. What makes this a great option is that they have unsaturated fats: the kind that you want. Specifically, nuts have polyunsaturated fats, just like olive oil. Walnut is one such example of a food with this healthy fat. You don't have to worry about the calories for nuts either, because for the healthy ones like walnuts, they usually end up being insignificant.

I don't want to spend too much time on vegetables because everyone knows that we are supposed to eat vegetables, but I will give you one more reason to eat them: they are packed with fiber. Of course, fiber aids in digestion. When you combine your fiber from your vegetable-rich diet with intermittent fasting, your digestive system will be as healthy as it can be. Fiber is also great for IF because it keeps you from feeling hungry during your fasting periods.

Avocados seem to be quite popular these days, but they really should be with IF practitioners. They are considered a "superfood" because they have a lot of the vitamins and nutrients that you need every day. Best of all, they have unsaturated fats. You can start eating a lot of avocados and get a lot of what you need from them so you can lower your caloric consumption.

While green tea may have chemicals that directly influence the power of autophagy, other teas could help with aspects of IF from a more pragmatic standpoint. For instance, while caffeine has been shown to help increase autophagy when it is generated, if you get that caffeine from coffee, it will also help you feel fuller. Coffee or any kind of tea may have this effect on you.

Eat eggs, too. They have the protein that you need without a lot of the unhealthy stuff that tends to come with protein. And while we are talking about studies, there is research showing that people who replace a bagel with an egg feel less feelings of hunger during the day — so you might want to get into the habit of eating an egg every morning so you can have the best chances of succeeding with IF.

There you have it — the foods to eat and to leave out when you do IF. You can always check this chapter again if you're unsure what to do, but you should also learn to trust your instinct about what foods to eat.

You feel one way after eating a bag of Skittles and another after Brussels sprouts. You know which one is going to help you get these positive health effects, and you know which one will hinder you.

Beware the tricks your mind will play on you to make you think that you are hungry for foods that do not even have essential nutrients. You can be sure this is just your brain trying to get the food you crave into your mouth.

Many people start the very first few hours into a fast and are convinced that they are already low on energy. True fatigue is one thing, but feeling a little tired after not eating for a couple of hours doesn't mean you need to eat a meal right away. You have to let feelings like this pass, or else they will seriously hinder your fast.

You are bound to feel like you are "slightly hungry" during your time doing the IF. This is something that you should expect with any fast after you spend your whole life never even contemplating it. Just be sure to know the difference between discomfort and pain — between unhealthy and "no pain, no gain."

Chapter 6

Intermittent Fasting and Women

There is good reason to learn about intermittent fasting specifically as it applies to women because research has demonstrated that it has different effects on men and women. This is because women studied exhibited some less-than-desirable outcomes as a result of intermittent fasting. I tell you this to caution you about doing it in a healthy way, not to scare you from doing something that would be good for your body.

Some women said their menstrual cycle altered because of it, and some said their blood sugar went too low. Both of these outcomes can be avoided by consuming adequate nutrients when you are not fasting and by limiting your fasting times to reasonable windows.

All the success that women have been having with IF is the reason that it has gotten so popular suddenly. It's a pattern of eating that speaks to the health concerns that women are worried about: weight loss, risk of heart disease, risk of diabetes, and even risk of cancer.

While any person can do it, you know that women have their own specific issues that make their experience with IF different. But how exactly do their experiences differ?

It is just one study on laboratory mice, but there is one that showed that female mice who did concurrent day fasting for 3-6 had ovaries that were shrunk and irregular cycles, too.

One way is in the menstrual cycle and how it can interact with changes in diet. There has not been any scientific backing yet on if intermittent fasting can really affect your period, but there has definitely been a limited number of cases where women say their cycles were different, and they thought that IF was the cause.

It is hard to say if we can blame this entirely on the IF routine itself, though. Some have suggested that since women who do it often want to lose weight, they are more likely to be overweight or obese. Being overweight or obese is a risk factor for having irregular periods, so perhaps this is the cause of the irregular cycle. However, we can't jump to conclusions.

But the menstrual cycle is not the only thing that women have to consider when doing IF that men don't. Their hormones are also different and affecting their eating habits differently.

These hormone differences give some credence to the idea that this diet can have negative consequences for women if you are not careful. The main hormone in the spotlight is GnRH, which is affected when women consume fewer calories.

If women consume too few calories, their GnRH might be interrupted, which could put them at risk for irregular periods.

We do have to keep in mind that this is a side effect of low caloric intake, not IF. Women who want to lose weight, to some extent, do just have to consume fewer calories. These women may accept the temporary changes to their period, knowing that their weight loss will have many positive, long-lasting benefits.

There may still be something to the idea that women should think about their specific issues when choosing to do this diet. They might choose to fast for a shorter period of time and for fewer days.

If we are being honest, while anyone can do an intermittent fast to get the health benefits of autophagy, most of the people who are doing it are women. The science showing women some of the woman-specific problems that come with it shouldn't scare them from doing it. They should keep doing it anyway because the initial discomfort is worth the payoff they will get when they lose weight, have better skin, and have a detoxified system.

Doctors know that women have reproductive systems that are closely related to their metabolisms. This makes sense because when women are carrying children, they have to be able to feed them from the inside.

Even if you aren't pregnant, however, the deep entanglement between the female reproductive system and the female metabolism affects your body. When you have not had a period for a while during the same time that you changed your pattern of eating, there is a greater-than-luck chance that your missing period is because of your fasting.

You don't want to give up on fasting just because it can be hard as a woman. You need to take the challenge and do the thing that is good for your body, even when it puts you through some periods of discomfort.

Remember that hormone changes are fleeting, so if you experience a change in hormones during the time that you fast, it doesn't mean that the fast is bad for you. Over time, they will adjust until it is just another part of your day.

Getting used to it will be a matter of managing your stress and sleep. Mostly, you want to pay attention to your stress, but your stress is connected to a whole list of things. They include not eating enough calories, not getting enough nutrients, not being active enough, chronic inflammation, and finally, sleep deprivation.

If you can manage all of these things, your hormones should not give you too much of a trouble as you transition into IF.

Nonetheless, going for an extended period of time without a period could be a sign of something serious. If this happens, you should stop your fast and schedule a doctor's visit.

Intermittent Fasting and Women: Made for Each Other

Don't let the anecdotal stories about irregular cycles make you afraid of doing what will ultimately be good for you. If you are being honest with yourself, at least part of the reason you would think IF could be harmful to women is so you don't have to do the work to get autophagy's benefits.

In all truth, autophagy is a wonderful way that women can take control of their bodies. Every woman on Earth wants a sustainable way to lose weight, increase muscle mass, and rev up their energy. Women that generate autophagy with intermittent fasting comes with all of these rewards, so it's no wonder so many women are talking about it.

As you know well, autophagy also confers long-term health benefits, but some of them are particularly important to women: a more acute stress response from their cells so that it is easier to trigger in the future, improved sensitivity to insulin, and an increase in the growth hormone, which is vital to many processes that your body goes through.

With all of these positives from IF, it wouldn't be wise to completely ignore some of the indications that it can interfere with the female reproductive system, too. But that only means we need to be measured in the way we generate autophagy. It doesn't mean we abandon IF altogether.

I am not saying that women should never do a full, 24-hour extended water fast. However, if you ever experience any signs that this diet influences your cycle, then it might be a good idea to avoid that long of a fast. It might be better for you to fast for around 12 hours instead.

Since you don't yet know how your body will react to fasting as a woman until you have done it, I also advise you to start very slow with your first fast. You probably should not even fast for two days in a row during your first week, if you really want to be careful.

There are some groups of women that should not do the aforementioned diet altogether. If you have had a history of problems with any major organs, such as your lungs, heart, or liver, you should not do it. It could put too much stress on these organs, and the potential benefit you would get from it would not be enough to justify you harming them.

It should be obvious that pregnant women should not fast. As I have said, the female reproductive system is closely tied to the woman's metabolism. When that woman is with child, she doesn't have the luxury of purposefully depriving herself of nutrients to generate autophagy anymore, because now the health of her body and of her child is what determines her health the most.

Sadly, there are many women with eating disorders compared to men. Women who have or who have had eating disorders should not attempt to do this diet. They are at too high a risk of losing any progress they might have made in establishing normal eating patterns.

My final two tips for women who do it are the same ones I have said throughout our book: drink a lot of water and exercise. Both of these activities will keep your body in shape so it can handle the stress of autophagy and IF better.

Chapter 7:

Intermittent Fasting for Women over 50

Overweight women over 50 have a higher risk of diabetes and heart problems than they did when they were younger. IF is one option they have to manage their weight and control these health risks.

The metabolism of a woman over 50 has become slower, so you can't expect quick results if you are a member of this group, but you will probably get the most out of it than any other group of women because of all the anti-aging effects of IF and autophagy.

Overweight and obese people have higher risks of heart disease, stroke, and more as they age. On the other hand, thinner people are not looking at these same risks.

Losing weight can only be good for your body, and autophagy is the healthiest and most effective way to do it, as it will help you stay thin, feel good, and be healthy for years and years.

But, so far, we have only talked about the health benefits that are immediately obvious. There is also a reduction of health risks that are not cosmetic like youthful skin and weight loss. It has been proven that an increase in the aforementioned phenomenon reduces your risk of Alzheimer's and Parkinson's disease.

Furthermore, it also reduces inflammation, which will increase your overall health. There has even been research about the benefits for cancer patients undergoing chemotherapy.

Studies have shown that cancer patients going through chemotherapy saw a reduction in the clumps of white blood cells that accumulate because of it. Dead cells can be hazardous to your body if they are not cleaned out during autophagy.

Since these patients fasted in order to turn on autophagy, their bodies were able to clean out the white blood cells and recover from chemotherapy sooner.

You can only imagine the kind of advantage you get if you are turning it on as much as possible, and you aren't even looking at a major health risk yet. You may not have as big an accumulation of dead cells as someone going through chemotherapy, but if you have not fasted before and you don't exercise regularly, it is very likely that you have a lot of toxins in your body.

This is because if you don't go through it very often, materials like dead cells, dead organelles, and unused proteins start to pile up and make your cells less efficient.

Putting your body through it doesn't just combat aging in ways that are immediately visible. It also greatly reduces your risk of long-term age-related disease. Whether you're looking to improve the quality of your life or the length of your life, making it happen in your body will do it.

There are many misconceptions about how the process does its anti-aging work. Perhaps the most common is that its only health benefits come from taking care of toxins. Clearing toxins from your system is certainly a good thing, but it goes far beyond ridding your body of harmful chemicals.

Most of these toxins are not from outside your body, but they are materials like proteins and organelles that your cells used once and then no longer had a use for. These discarded materials start to take up space over time, creating clutter that slows down your cells. This is when they become toxins.

Some of these toxins cause even worse problems than congestion. The worst case is protein clusters that form in the brain. Neurodegenerative diseases like Alzheimer's become more of a concern as we age, and autophagy might be your best ally in fighting against your risk of these diseases.

From a broader perspective, Alzheimer's manifests as "knots" and "tangles" in the brain that impair memory.

When doctors look at the knots and tangles with a microscope, they see that these irregularities are actually clusters of proteins that have built up over time. They are proteins that brain cells used at one point but later had no purpose. The protein clusters were not managed with autophagy, so they simply accumulated and started leading to serious memory problems.

Alzheimer's disease is the most extreme consequence that you can have from not going through enough autophagy. It is not the only consequence, however. Discarded materials like protein clusters start to build up throughout your body if you rarely go through this process.

In this regard, low autophagy leads to a low count of collagen, the protein that makes your skin youthful. Your skin cells can't produce collagen when they are crowded by cellular garbage.

Similarly, you lose more muscle mass if you rarely go through it because you are not turning on it to repair the muscle tissue damage that results from physical activity.

From these examples alone, you can see that this phenomenon is more than a toxin-cleaning agent, as it doesn't only destroy the bad (toxins); it builds the good (new organelles, proteins, and cells). Both sides of it make it such a powerful anti-aging tool, one that was surprisingly given to us by nature.

So far, we have established that it isn't just good for destroying pathogen invaders — it also destroys materials that become toxic when they linger in the cell for too long. In short, this biological process cleans out toxins from the outside and inside.

In the third stage, your cells use these broken-down parts as ingredients to build new cells and cell structures. What's more: your cells have more room to build new cells and new cell parts because they freed up so much space during autophagy.

All these things come together when you find a way to turn on it on a regular basis. Equipped with all this information, you know much more about this than even your average fasting practitioner.

Women over 50 certainly still want to manage their weight and have good skin, but it is around this age that we start to get a more mature perspective on life, and we care more about the health consequences of our daily life choices than before. They have many options for unlocking autophagy even further than they would with IF alone.

Back in the 90s, the idea of caloric restriction became very popular, and people saw improvements in their health from doing nothing more than eating less. There is even a great deal of evidence that mammals who restrict their calories live longer than mammals who do not.

This has not yet been proven to be true for humans, but still, restricting your caloric intake can only be a good thing. You get this additional benefit from turning on autophagy through fasting while also getting the benefit of autophagy itself along with it.

We have heard a lot of ideas about losing weight from nutritionists in the last few decades, but let's not kid ourselves: the main reason for weight gain across the planet comes down to people consuming a lot of calories without physically exerting themselves to burn them off. Fasting for any length of time will lead to consuming fewer calories, so you are on the right track for losing weight when you fast.

The next popular method of turning on it is the keto diet. This method will turn on autophagy because it involves depriving your body of nutrients that it would normally consume for energy.

However, following the keto diet alone will not turn on it because it is only activated when your cells are in a state of stress, and as long as you are sedentary or filling your body with any kind of food, your cells are not in this state.

That said, since the keto diet is so low in carbs, this style of eating will aid in turning on autophagy. I definitely recommend following the keto diet because the mistake many practitioners make is consuming a lot of carbs while they are not fasting.

Eating a lot of carbs will prevent your body from fasting for a long time because it takes a long time for your digestive system to process them. Not only that, but as you may be aware, it becomes harder to keep weight off the older you get, and you are significantly slowing down the process of burning fat when your digestive tract has a backlog of carbs. Fighting against this problem is the role of the keto diet in anti-aging and autophagy.

Next, there is the method of good old exercise. Studies have shown that resistance training, also known as strength training, is the most effective way of turning on the process, saying it is even more effective than fasting. The reason for this is that when you use your muscles, you are getting tiny tears in your muscle tissue that are repaired through autophagy.

The unfortunate thing is that exercising might be the last thing that people want to do, even though it is so good for their health. Like the other methods, exercise has its own health benefits that are separate.

Plenty of studies show that people who work out regularly have lower risks of all age-related illnesses, even those not related to the heart. If we are being honest, exercising is probably the best way to fight aging.

If you want to get the most out of autophagy, you should employ all of these methods together. When combined, the keto diet, exercise, and fasting will give you the greatest benefits, both in terms of weight loss and in general health.

If you don't yet feel motivated to be as healthy as possible, try to think of the autophagy in your cells as an analogy for your personal health. If they did not recycle their cellular garbage, your cells would simply die after their organelles stopped working or they were overcrowded with protein clusters and foreign invaders.

If you do not recycle your body's toxins by turning on autophagy regularly, your body will be over-encumbered with cellular garbage and you will be less healthy as a result. If this analogy were expanded, you might even live a shorter life if you do not regularly clean out your cellular garbage.

Your cells try to live longer by using this method to combat their cellular aging — you should try to use autophagy to work against aging too.

Chapter 8
Intermittent Fasting Techniques: 16/8, Keto Diet, and More

After talking a little bit about the different ways that women do intermittent fasting, and now it's time to go into them in detail. The first one, and maybe the most well-known, is the 16/8 one.

The fundamental aspect of IF — not eating for some period of the day — is easily observed in 16/8. You only eat for 8 hours of the day, and you fast for the other 16 hours. It is also typical for practitioners to follow the keto diet, a low-carb diet designed to induce ketosis in your body to help in burning body fat.

Many women get confused about what intermittent fasting requires of them because they are used to following diets, not fasts. It is a new pattern of eating, not a diet. There are foods that you should eat in an IF fast since they help with the goal of autophagy, as we learned in Chapter 5. But itself is not a diet.

The other side of that is women thinking they can eat anything since it is not a diet. This is obviously not true either.

In one sense, IF is simpler than dieting. You could say it's simpler because you are not basing all of your health and body goals on eating certain foods and restricting others. On a fundamental level, the most important thing to do for is to commit to not eating for a number of hours at the same time every day.

But you could also say that it is more complicated, because its advocates — me included — will not make the claim that fasting alone will do everything. The truth is, the IF itself is doing most of the work, but you will only see the results if you adopt habits that are good for your health, too.

That said, I hope this book has given you a good sense of how autophagy ties into all aspects of health, because it really does tie into intermittent fasting, working out, and eating healthy.

The point we are trying to come to is that you could work out every day and eat all of the foods you are supposed to eat, but not fast; you would be healthy, without a doubt. But on balance, you probably wouldn't be as healthy as someone who worked out a little less, ate a little less healthy, but did IF every day.

That's because autophagy is the vital cellular process your whole body relies upon, but that people do not pay nearly enough attention to.

You are nearing the end of the book, and that means it's time to put together your plan of attack for this fast. What kind are you going to do? Whichever one you choose, you should write down your exact goal for the number of hours you want to fast and the date you will start.

When the day comes, mark the actual time you start fasting and the actual time you stop. Write down whether you "cheat" during your fasting window or not. Keeping a log like this will make it a lot more likely for you to do it successfully.

The 12-Hour Fast

This intermittent fast is a good one to start with, although if the idea of fasting is completely new to you and makes you nervous, you are totally free to reduce it to 10 hours or less.

The trick for a simple intermittent fast like this is to ensure you are still getting the healthy number of calories every day but to simply get them outside of the 12-hour long window that you have decided to fast for.

The 12-hour fast is also a good place to start for someone who wants to end up doing a more ambitious fast. You don't start so low that going as high as 16 hours seems infeasible. You may even want to work up to a 20-hour fast if you are feeling bold, though, at that point, you may want to consider trying the 24-hour water fast.

The times during which you use the indicated approach are entirely up to you. Any approach is best done by waking up relatively early, eating breakfast, fasting, and then eating dinner not too soon before bed. You don't want to eat too close to your bedtime because then you will be spending a lot of your precious autophagy time during sleep by breaking down your food.

It is surprising that we have not even had the opportunity to talk about the importance of sleep with autophagy. There are some facts about sleep and it is that you need to seriously consider.

You do the most autophagy that you do throughout your day when you are sleeping. Even in people who do not think about fasting or autophagy whatsoever, their highest level of it is when they are sleeping, and so is yours.

That means when you eat really close to the time you go to bed — let's say you eat at 7pm and then sleep at 9pm — you aren't giving your body enough time to break down your food. You don't have any significant autophagy when you are digesting, so digesting in your sleep is a big wasted opportunity.

Even the 12-hour fast can prove challenging, because you don't want to wake up too unreasonably early, but you don't want to digest food during the time that you should be going through advanced autophagy while you are asleep, either.

You may choose to wake up and eat your first meal at 7am. 12 hours later, your fast is over, and you eat dinner at 7pm. You can probably already see how this can problematic; if you get enough sleep to wake up at 7am, you will want to be in bed by 10pm. However, this does leave 3 hours between your dinner and your bedtime, so while it is a tight squeeze, this system does work out for the 12-hour fast.

The 8-Hour Fast

You could call this a beginner fast. That doesn't mean that it's a small feat, though. Don't forget that IF is every day. 8 hours may not seem like a long time to go without food, but if you haven't done it before, doing it every day might end up being a lot harder than you expected.

Some call the 16-hour fast the "16:8 diet," so you can call this one the "8:16 diet," if you like. As you can see, leaving plenty of time between dinner and sleep is a lot easier with this diet. You can eat dinner at 6pm, go to bed at 10pm, wake up at 7am, and get your nutrients between then and 10am. But between 10am and 6pm, you are doing your intermittent fast.

It is funny how compared to the 12-hour fast the 8-hour fast seems like it is a small feat, but when you get down to what is expected, it is still a hard thing for many people to do — especially every day.

The 5:2 Fast

Not every kind of intermittent fasting is based around the number of hours you fast every day. In earnest, I recommend doing the traditional 8-hour fast to start out and simply make it longer as you become more comfortable. However, I have said throughout the book that you have the freedom to do whatever works for you and your body — so it would be a disservice to you if I didn't let you know what other options are out there for IF.

In 5:2, you eat the way you would normally for five days of the week (still eating healthy, though). During the other two days, women only consume 500 calories.

The usual guidance applies — you don't get to glut out on your non-fasting days just because you aren't in a fast. You will want to make sure you get all the nutrients you need on the non-fasting days, though, because you won't be able to cram many important ones into 500 calories on those days.

There are some people who think 5:2 would work better for them because they can't imagine committing to fasting every single day of the week. With 5:2, you do an extreme fast for two days of the week so that you don't have to fast at all on most days of the week.

Concurrent Day Fasting

This kind of fast itself has different versions to it, but they all follow the basic idea of fasting every other day instead of every single day. It is similar to the 5:2 fast, except you don't have to go as extreme on your fasting days.

Concurrent day fasting, sometimes called alternate day fasting, has been tested in some studies, and people did have luck in losing weight when following it. The main drawback of it is that people say they never feel entirely full when following it.

If you want to follow concurrent day fasting yourself, you don't have to do much to plan it out. Of course, you eat on whatever schedule you normally would on your non-fasting days, and then every other day you fast.

Since you aren't fasting every day, you need to consider that when deciding how long you will go. You don't want to do an 8-hour fast, because that is too short, considering that you will go back to not fasting the next day. A 12- or 16-hour fast might work, depending on your experience with it so far.

You have no shortage of options for IF. I hope you feel that thanks to this book, you are at no shortage of information, either.

You may feel somewhat overwhelmed after reading guide to intermittent fasting that is so chockfull of information. The Table of Contents may be helpful to you in case you think you should revisit a topic again.

Conclusion

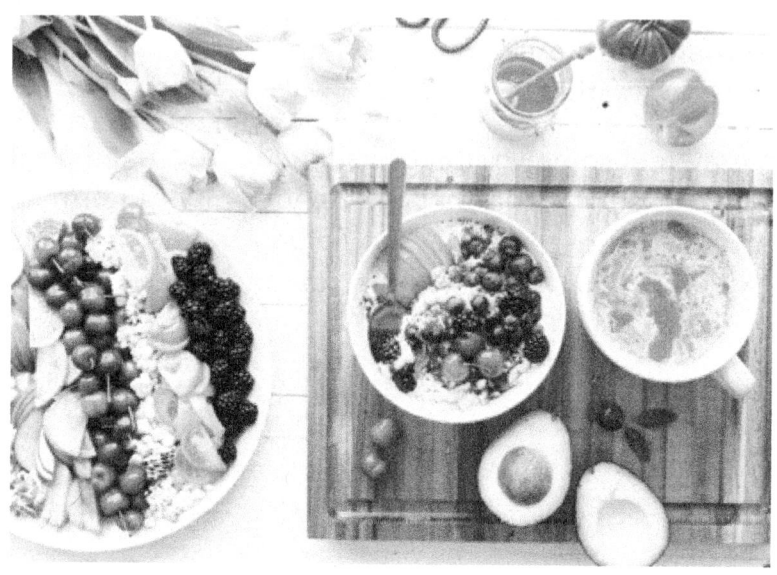

Thank you for making it through to the end of *Intermittent Fasting for Women 101*, let's hope it was informative and able to provide you with all of the tools you need to achieve your goals whatever they may be.

After being exposed to so much knowledge about intermittent fasting, you aren't likely to be surprised by the fact that the American Heart Association recommends it for losing weight. Its effectiveness in helping women lose weight is backed by science as well as by the personal experiences of thousands of women.

Fasting has existed in religious traditions for millennia, and now anyone can harness its health benefits with intermittent fasting. You don't have to undergo nearly the level of physical and mental fatigue of traditional water fasts, but you still see the difference in your waistline and in how you feel.

The scientific credibility that IF has is all thanks to the biological process of autophagy. Autophagy is your body's natural means of getting rid of toxins that pollute your system. Intermittent fasting is your means of triggering this vital process.

Biologists have been studying autophagy and its revelatory implications for health heavily in the last ten years — and some of the most important findings have been in just the last few years! Be sure to check out the appendix at the end of the book so you can learn more about what scientists are finding out.

The more and more mainstream attention that autophagy has been receiving can be attributed to the research of Nobel Prize-winning Yoshinori Ohsumi. He is the scientist who studied it in yeast cells for decades and was finally recognized for his important work.

His research led to more scientists studying the role of this process in fighting cancer and age-related disease. What has been found is that triggering it on purpose can help us live healthier lives, longer lives, and more youthful lives.

Intermittent fasting is your ticket into triggering autophagy because it is easy to sustain. Unlike other means of achieving autophagy, intermittent fasting doesn't ask that you go to the gym or change what you eat (although you should still these things to get the most out of the biological process). Start your intermittent fast today and you will see all the health benefits uncovered in this book for yourself.

If you're still skeptical, make sure to peruse the appendix, which is filled with scientific studies on intermittent fasting done by experts.

Finally, if you found this book useful in any way, a review on Amazon is always appreciated

Appendix: **Studies on Intermittent Fasting and Autophagy**

Anton, Moehl, Donahoo, Marosi, Lee, et al. *Flipping the Metabolic Switch: Understanding and Applying Health Benefits of Fasting*. 2017 Oct 31.

ncbi.nlm.nih.gov/pmc/articles/PMC5783752/

This study focuses on the physical effects of intermittent fasting on the most important organs of the body. The authors conclude that lowering the level of glucose in your body can actually aid in keeping your muscle mass. They say this can be a boon for people who are struggling with their weight. They even conclude that fasting results in the activation of neural pathways with a lot of great effects, in including fighting aging and slow the progression of disease.

Bartosz, Zalewska, Wesierska, Sokolowska, et al. *Intermittent Fasting in Cardiovascular Disorders—An Overview*. Published 2019 Mar 20.

ncbi.nlm.nih.gov/pmc/articles/PMC6471315/

The authors conclude that doing intermittent fasting greatly reduces the risk of getting a cardiovascular disease. Participants in this eating pattern are able to maintain a source of energy through fatty acids and ketones while the body goes through metabolic switching between glucose and ketones. These scientists even conclude that intermittent fasting helps people lose body mass by changing the transformations of your lipids. They also say that it reduces cholesterol in its practitioners.

Antunes, Erustes, Costa, Nascimento, et al. *Autophagy and intermittent fasting: the connection for cancer therapy?* Published 2018 Nov 27.

ncbi.nlm.nih.gov/pmc/articles/PMC6257056/

These authors examine the role that autophagy can play in fighting against cancer. They write that this phenomenon can either help cancer cells grow or help non-cancerous cells grow to fight against them, depending on the situation. They consider the possible use of autophagy for fighting tumors. Fasting in particular is outlined as the chief strategy in using autophagy to fight cancer. The main conclusion is the use of it for protecting non-cancerous cells from toxic cancer cells as well as for reducing the side effects from chemotherapy.

Ganesan, Habboush, Sultan. *Intermittent Fasting: The Choice for a Healthier Lifestyle.* Published online 2018 Jul 9. ncbi.nlm.nih.gov/pmc/articles/PMC6128599/

A meta-analysis of studies done in the past 20 years on the subject of intermittent fasting. Not only did these studies show that people who did intermittent fasting lost weight, but they also improved on important biological measures like reduced low-density lipoprotein and triglyceride. No matter the body type of the studies' participants, they succeeded in losing weight on average.

Harvie, Howell. *Potential Benefits and harms of Intermittent Energy Restriction and Intermittent Fasting Amongst Obese, Overweight and Normal Weight Subjects—A Narrative Review of Human and Animal Evidence.* Published 2017 Jan 19.

ncbi.nlm.nih.gov/pmc/articles/PMC5371748/

These authors go over and compare experiments on intermittent fasting and intermittent energy restriction (referred to in this book as caloric restriction). Their findings are that there is no real evidence of either method being harmful, and while both methods show promise for helping people lose weight, fasting is more consistently effective. They note that there is a lack of research on the effective of intermittent fasting and caloric restriction on people who are not overweight or obese.

Jacomin, Gul, Sudhakar, Korcsmaros, Nezis. *What We Learned from Big Data for Autophagy Research.* Published 2018 Aug 17.

ncbi.nlm.nih.gov/pmc/articles/PMC6107789/

The scientists went into this study wanting to investigate the relation between autophagy and other integral cellular processes. They use big data to do an overview of what biologists have learned about this relation. The authors find that autophagy plays an important part in many different pathologies, including in infections and in cancer. Its role in neurodegenerative diseases is also well-known.

Yoshii, Mizushima. *Monitoring and Measuring Autophagy.* 2017 Sep 18.

ncbi.nlm.nih.gov/pmc/articles/PMC5618514/

Yoshii and Mizushima examine a number of meta issues in studying autophagy, including the use of mice and their anatomical closeness to humans and the accuracy of the results in studies that use samples to make conclusions about autophagy in human beings.

Intermittent Fasting Diet Guide

*A Complete Step-By-Step Guide for Heal
Your Body, Weight Loss, Fat Burn and Live
in a Healthy and Happy Way with
the Autophagy Process
(Meal Plan with 60 Recipes).*

Jennifer Cook

Introduction

Losing weight, getting in shape and a healthy lifestyle is all what we need nowadays. Many people out there are looking for the best options that can help them to be in a good shape and manage weight. In order to achieve the required results, people are using a number of tricks and following tips. In the weight management industry, though, there is a number of trends coming up for anyone who wants to have the best shape and body type.

If you want to lose weight the very first thing that comes on your list is diet, of course; it is known that you need to cut down your food intake. Some people strongly believe in this trick while others do not. Some fitness freaks believe in taking food of good quality and doing exercise properly. They claim that with proper workout and exertion you will be able to cut down the fats and reduce weight.

In general, both claims are good enough. As a matter of fact, these tricks and tips work amazingly for people who persistently used them. However, in some scenarios, all these methods do have some reactions on people: for instance, some are not good enough with workout and weights, so they may collapse. Differently, others opt some hardcore dieting that cause them to lack some of the essential minerals in the body.

To be in good shape and follow a healthy pattern it is necessary to employ some of the safe and recommended solutions. Only diet or exercise are not acceptable, so it is necessary to combine them with methods that actually work. Exercise never refers to hitting the gym; if you are doing any physical activity, it means that you have an exercise arrangement in your routine. Moreover, dieting never asks you not to eat, but to eat properly.

Other than these methods, there is the fasting method. This approach helps you to make a major difference in your overall appearance and fitness plan. All you need is to ensure what kind of fasting you are going to start. Here in this book, it is written everything about the intermittent fasting: its types, tricks and diet options. It is a complete package for you to get started today and observe your results.

Chapter 1
Intermittent Fasting

On your way to a healthy and balanced life with a well-toned body, you came across with so many options. If you want to go for something that will help you in a long run without damaging health, then intermittent fasting can be the choice. It is something that keeps your lifestyle balanced: it surely helps you to avoid taking the heavy and junk food options and it makes you sure to digest everything you eat.

Commonly, we put on weight because the food we ingest is not digesting perfectly. When our food is perfectly digested, we will be able to make a visible change in ourselves. Fasting is one of the helpful ways to make you digest food properly in a balanced manner, in order to have the best nutrients from food. It will not let the fats and energy stored in the body as well; in fact, all the contents of our diet are digested and utilized correctly in our body.

What Is Fasting?

Before getting into the intermittent fasting, it is necessary to understand the concept of it. Most of the people relate it to starving and keeping the stomach empty for long hours. It is a considerable fact that fasting is not just about keeping the stomach empty or starves for no reason. In some part of the world people fast as a religious obligation while, some of them, use it as a method to be in shape and lose weight.

Studies show that to achieve the better health standard, it is necessary for a person to keep the stomach empty for about 10 to 12 hours. It helps a person to make the use of all the body fats and ensure the complete utilization of the energy. Generally, we are unable to hit the empty stomach because we take the meals after intervals. In these intervals, our food is not able to digest and burn properly in the body.

However, with fasting things change and they are quite different. When a person fasts for almost 12 hours, it burns the stored fuel inside; this helps to reach an empty stomach and some extra fuel used from the reserves. Overall, it is helpful to have a balanced and attractive body.

Systematic procedure

It is a notable fact that fasting is not a random act that one can do on his/her own. A systematic procedure needs to be design according to a pattern. The use of patterns helps a person to hit the right results. In case, if you do a random fasting, you will face the consequences, not the result for the effort. So, make sure you are going to have enough knowledge about the fasting, its techniques and other important details.

What Is Intermittent Fasting?

Intermittent fasting is becoming a trendy way to lose weight. It is considered the best way to slim down in short time. Besides that, it is also improving metabolic health and even extending the lifespan. The most amazing part of intermittent fasting is that it has a few methods. You can opt the one that suits you.

Losing weight is not an issue now. You just need to make up your mind and need some courage. Select any method from the intermittent fasting methods, as all the approaches are effective and they will give you promising results.

Intermittent fasting is an eating schedule: it alternates eating and fasting. You set a period of eating according to your goal and after setting the eating time, you have to stick to it. Remember to eat only during eating hours and fast for the rest of the hours.

In the past, it was used to treat people suffering from obesity, diabetes, and epilepsy. Now it is used to lose weight and it is a healthy method that helps your body to function in a better way.

Intermittent Fasting And Weight Loss

We have discussed that intermittent fasting have been used for multiple purposes: it has been a treatment for some health problems and issues that includes diabetes, epilepsy and even obesity. Intermittent fasting is one of the ancient and known method that helped a number of people to slim down and get a healthy lifestyle.

While you are looking into the weight loss journey from the point of intermittent fasting, the procedure is quite clear and normal; there is no science involved in it. The only thing that comes in, is the schedule and a complete routine chart so, once a person is doing it right, he/she will get the best results.

How Intermittent Fasting Helps To Lose Weight?

Usually, in weight loss and management, the professionals do not recommend to starve your body; they have methods to help you increase your metabolism and manage the overall diet to ensure the best outcomes. However, in case of intermittent fasting, things are quite different and advanced: the professionals suggest you to try the fasting in order to get rid of extra fats from the body. The fasting is not random but a systematic procedure that eventually helps you to achieve the right size. Here is a procedure that you need to follow:

Start with the short intervals

To achieve the right results from intermittent fasting, it is important to start with the short intervals. We need to make our body familiar with the feeling of fasting. It is helpful to make things easy to digest and appealing for the body as well. If you start up with the long intervals, you may not be able to get the desired results, as they will directly cause you to lose the energy levels and you will not be able to perform the daily task. Make sure that you are going to train the body first, and then will lead things to the larger limits in getting the problem sorted.

Never leave the stomach empty but make it empty

Intermitting fasting is not about starving or keeping your stomach empty. In fact, it works on a better and rapid metabolism by letting the stomach to use all the food in it and consume energy from it till the end. It is possible when you take short meals and the interval between them is longer than usual. It helps the stomach to work

252

properly and get the best energy out of the food portion that you have taken in a specific time.

Using the stored energy

Through intermittent fasting, you can remove fats by using them in regular work. It is obvious that you need some energy to perform tasks. That energy comes from the food we eat or fuel we have stored in the body. When we eat something, we consume the energy that is required and the rest of it gets stored in the body, and lastly it becomes fats. To reduce weight and fats it is necessary to get rid of that stored fat from the body. In this scenario, the important thing is to breakdown fats again in the useable energy and gets them out from the body.

In the procedure of intermittent fasting, the body gets into the position to disintegrate the stored fats energy in the body and then consumes it. Although it takes time, it really works and it gets you to the easiest way out to reduce weight.

Chapter 2
Intermittent Fasting Benefits

"Health is your future investment to live
a balanced life with all profits."
Unknown

The method of intermittent fasting is not popular because it is in trend. In fact, this is something exceptional that actually helps a person to clear many problems. It is not just the weight loss that is achieved from the fasting, but there are also a number of benefits that we cannot measure. For a healthy, prosperous and balanced life, it is one of the best and possibly effective strategies. This method does not focus on your body shape, but it supports the other organs and overall body structure too.

Unlike other methods of healthy living and weight loss, fasting makes you even stronger: not just about a lighter body but its purification and health that last for long. It is good to find out about the ultimate benefits of the intermittent fasting, therefore you can do it by heart and you will know what you are going to get out of it.

How Intermittent Fasting Helps?

Most of the people question how intermittent fasting can help you to lose weight or purify the body; the answer is simple. When you have calculated intake of food with a guided chart, then you will be using the other possible and healthy options to keep the balance of your body. A systematic procedure works in specific intervals to let your body release all the toxins, and it improves the body immunity as well.

Purification of the body

This process helps you to purify the body and organs as well. When we take a meal for the first 8 hours and then we fast for the next 16 hours in a day, it means that we will take the selective food only. The food should be something that takes time to digest and provides us the energy, gradually. Moreover, during the fasting timings, we will focus on the detox water, herbal tea or other electrolytes to maintain the glucose level. The selection of food will definitely exclude the fast food and energy drinks from the diet. In the end, we will be relying on the natural options like fruits, whole wheat and vegetables; it will help to boost the metabolism and reduce the overall toxins.

Structural transformation

Fasting supports you to make some of the amazing structural transformations. It is not just about the fat reduction but to get the muscle definition and structure designing. If you want to be in a specific body shape, with the help of the intermittent fasting and workout, you can make a real difference in your appearance too. Both factors together support you to sustain a position that you always wanted to have.

Inner cleansing

For a healthy and presentable personality, we mainly focus on the outer cleansing that starts from the apparels to the skin. However, to sustain the personality you should have inner cleansing that purifies your organs and keeps your blood clean as well. Intermittent fasting plays an integral role in cleansing your body from inside that leaves and impact on every cell and its formation too. From the blood cells to the tissues and even organs, it makes everything clean and purified in your body. However, this purification is directly linked with your routine and the food intake you are having in the period. Make sure that you are not going to compromise the routine and you are following the best diet plan for the intermittent fasting. It will make you get the desired results in the end.

Healthy organs

Due to our poor diet management and lifestyle, we commonly face a number of health issues and problems. Kidney stone, liver issues, diabetes, heart problems, hypertension, and so on. All these issues are related to the poor performing organs in our body. These organs are mostly under threat, due to careless diet plans and poor weight management as well. With the support of intermittent fasting, we can make our organs healthy and take care of the essentials that keep up running in our life. Studies evaluate that people following healthy diet with intermittent fasting, have organs with better health and do not face much health related issues. In fact, it helps them to recover any damage happened to the organs by keeping the things in control and scheduled.

Better immune system

Most of the problems that come up to our body is due to weak immune system; it increases the chances of infections and bacterial attacks. Intermittent fasting is not just limited to the weight control or organ purification. In fact, it is linked with the overall immune system and body balance.

Health Benefits

It is not possible to evaluate and record the health benefits of intermittent fasting. Intermittent fasting has a number of benefits that cover up multiple dimensions, so we cannot conclude any specific benefits. However, it overall makes you feel healthy and cover up some of the critical health issues for you. Here are some direct benefits that you can get from the intermittent fasting.

Treating diabetes

People suffering from the diabetes can use this method to keep their glucose level in blood controlled and avoid any other issues. For them it is important to take care of what they eat and how they eat. Everything is related to total consumption and its reaction to the people. With the help of intermittent fasting, a diabetic can actually enhance the overall immunity levels and make visible changes in the diabetic conditions.

Rescue Alzheimer

We all are afraid of losing anything, no matter if are money, things or even memories; we do not want to take risk with anything. Nonetheless, Alzheimer is one of the diseases that takes gradually all the memories from our brain away. It is not a sudden problem but with the passage of time it causes trouble in cognition, coordination and retention of the information as well. Intermittent fasting is one of the solutions to help a person with Alzheimer, as long as it enables the body and mind to fight against the disorder and secure the memories from being completely lost.

Fat and weight reduction

Another major benefit that has made the intermittent fasting popular is the weight and fat reduction from the body. The logic is simple, when you are taking limited meals for a specific time, you consequently are taking limited calories. However, all your activities are on the same page, so you are consuming more calories than your intake; finally, it will put a direct effect on your body, weight and fat layers.

Better metabolism

When you are not overloading your stomach with a lot of food and giving it time to work properly in time to digest it, then you are working to improve your metabolism. Eventually the stomach will be able to digest and process food properly; this will help you to get all the nutrients absorbed properly in blood and take all the benefits from it. Moreover, it will encourage you to avoid any kind of stomach problems, as your food is completely digested.

Clean blood flow

During the fasting hours, as per schedule you need to take water, electrolytes and herbal teas that help you to clean up blood. The more we drink water, the more we detox, to finally get the blood purified. Moreover, it increases the blood flow to the whole body and in every organ as well. The better blood flow helps all the cells to receive the oxygenated blood and makes them healthy. Overall, you will get the best body health from the inside out. As a matter of fact, better blood flow helps the skin to breath, it makes it tighten and bright as well; therefore, you will not only get a good body shape but radiant skin too.

Proper organ functioning

Once you have better blood circulation to all the organs, providing them nutrient, proper rest, and exercises, it means that your overall health is getting better. It will make these organs function properly and you will get the best of lifestyle.

Reduce stress

Other than the body health benefits, this approach helps you to get rid of the psychological problems as well. The ultimate diet plan with a balanced exercise can help you to deal with the psychological stress problems. Good food and healthy lifestyle make you feel relax and let out all the negativity that reduces stress and makes your life peaceful.

Intermittent Fasting & Obesity

Intermittent fasting and obesity have a strong connection to each other: it is one of the appropriate solutions for all obese people. The fasting offers you multiple strategies to maintain and manage diet plans and meal intake. This ultimate range gives you the benefits of selection, as per preferences and adjustment. The meal strategy helps you to ensure the ultimate treatment to your obesity and it also helps you to manage it.

The ultimate solution

If a person selects the diet plans to reduce weight, then cravings are the worst enemy of that person. Getting stick to a strict diet plan is a hard choice for anyone. A person needs to cheat and have some other relaxation as well. On the other hand, hitting the gym is not possible for everyone. There are issues with strength, timings and dedication as well. Therefore, a person is left with the intermittent fasting; it is the only solution that lets a person to eat what he/she likes, works out a little and loses weight in real numbers. With fasting, you can take the meal in the meal hours and the rest is your fasting time, so you will have time to consume the energy you have taken in the meal.

Long-term results

Intermittent fasting is not like the other options of diet plans or gym. Any skip from these options will cost you much and you will get back to the previous shape. Instead, it lets you to have the long-term results. You will not put the weight on back until you are not careless about your regular intake. Moreover, it will become your routine that you will love to prolong.

Easy going and routine procedure

Following this meal plan approach and skipping is not a difficult task. You have the option to decide the calorie intake and you can shift from one strategy to the others. It overall helps you to maintain a cycle and stick to the lifestyle; it will not bother you much or you will not strive to quit it as soon as possible.

No side effects

Intermittent fasting has no side effects, unless you are not taking things for granted. A few things need to be considered for sure. You are not supposed to skip the meals for more than 16 hours. If you are skipping the meal for long, you need to take the calories in other meals accordingly, so you will not be drained. You need to take the electrolytes, exercise and water along with some fruits in your fast timings to keep the energy level in the body. Overall, if you are following a good schedule there is no side effect on your side.

Time is the key element

If you think that with intermittent fasting you will be able to feel the results quickly, then you are wrong. Expecting the magical results within no time is the issue. Commonly we become unsettled, when it comes to follow the results. In the intermittent fasting time is the key element that costs you. We do not put on weight within day, it takes weeks and months. The same thing happens when we are trying to dissolve fats and reduce weight; it will take months and sometimes year as well to get the visible results. It is important to consider that you need to keep practicing the routine without any break and you will get the results in time.

Know the body differences

The body type of every person is not the same. Some people have soft fats that are dissolved easily in less time, while others have hard fats that take time. Therefore, you need to know the body difference in the first place, so you can have the right results; this helps you to make your strategy accordingly and will take things forward as well. All you need is to determine your body type and except results as per your case. Do not fall into the trap of someone else's experience, as they are different from you.

Chapter 3
Who Can Do Fasting?

We know a lot about the intermittent fasting and we can understand that it is one of the ultimate solutions to many problems. However, we need to understand that it is a limited-edition solution that is available for some specific people. We cannot generalize the application or adaptation of the intermittent fasting, as it can have multiple effects.

Intermittent fasting is all about managing your meals and whole day activities. The need for meal for a day activity can be different from one person to another, one age to another and even in genders. In this regard, it is necessary to identify whether a person is eligible for intermittent fasting or not. Things can be tricky but it is not hard to evaluate whether you need to look into it or not. Here is a schedule where is explained who can do intermittent fasting or not.

Guide For Kids

There is no doubt that intermittent fasting is one of the efficient tools in weight management and obesity control. However, there is not enough evidence available to make it safe for the kids in their growing age. Kids and adolescents are in their growing age and they need the best of nutrients; they have a routine that involves physical exertion, learning new things and consuming energy, so they need to have regular meals, snacks and even some healthy options in their meal plan. Intermittent fasting can cause a barrier in the nutritional acquisition of these kids; therefore, to give them a healthy and balance life it is necessary to focus on their diet in the growing age.

The studies show that it is not a good idea to put your kid on intermittent fasting in his growing age. If the child is obese or need some weight or diet management, then many other options to help the child are available. Other than intermittent fasting, you can follow these tips:

Plan all the meals

There is the best way to plan up the meals for your kids: you need to keep the meal time and snack time specifically adjusted, so the kids will get everything on time; moreover, you need to manage the portion for everything, in order to get the balanced nutrients.

Purify the intake

The energy drinks, sugar beverages, cold drinks, excessive sweets, processed foods and junk foods cause obesity in kids as well. You need to purify their intake to the maximum and incorporate fresh fruits, vegetables and all healthy food items to their meal plan. Doing so, it will help them to get all the natural minerals and grow solid.

Promote mindful eating

Most of the kids lack at the mindful eating: it is about when the kid is eating with intention and attention. It is not good to force a kid to have a meal when is not mindful eating, or when he/she is playing game or watching TV with his/her meal. The kid should focus on the food and he/she should enjoy every bite of it. The strategy can help the kid to fell the taste and get full after the meal.

Mealtime is family time

Make sure to serve your kids a meal with family: they should sit together with the family and eat properly. It encourages them to finish their food with concentration and it will develop a sense of discipline to them.

Intermittent Fasting And Women

Intermittent fasting for men and women has a different approach. It is not necessary that both genders have different effects of the meal plans and fasting. For women it is important to consider whether the plan is suitable for them or not. There can be multiple reactions they could face for to intermittent fasting. The routine we develop do have a direct effect and impact on our hormonal balance, moods and psychological cognition as well.

Females are commonly considered as sensitive people, when it comes to react against the hormonal or diet changes. Therefore, for women it is necessary to assess their potential, in the first place, and then pick up the right meal plan for them.

Ideal plans for women

We cannot rationalize the meal plan and ideas for men and women in the intermittent fasting. Both have different needs, demands and reaction to the things. Thus, it is important to pay attention to their needs and possible reaction when designing a meal plan. Here we have some ideal plans for women that can help them to get the quick and fruitful results from the intermittent fasting. These plans come with a minimum risk of reaction or problems for female. The plans are designed according to the needs, reactions and body types of female in general.

Eat – stop – eat

A 24 hours protocol incorporates food intake two times a day with an interval of 14 to 16 hours in a cycle of 24 hours. For women, it is recommended twice a week and not more than that.

Crescendo method

It includes the fasting for about 12 to 16 hours for 2 or 3 nonconsecutive days in a week. It is important to spread the weeks evenly across the week.

5:2 diets

It is all about to restrict your calories to 25% for 2 days in a week and these can be two consecutive or nonconsecutive days as well. The rest of the days is normal to intake calories.

You can select any of the plans from the above-mentioned resources. However, all you need is to care about whether the plan suits you or not. It is important to find out whether you are comfortable with this meal plan or not. To try out what is appropriate for you, you can have the trial for short time and, if it suits you, then you can take the plan further, otherwise try another one.

Pregnancy is a no intermittent fasting zone

During pregnancy, women are restricted to try intermittent fasting. In the reproduction, state female needs to have multi nutrients and a complete supply of food and minerals that help in the fetus development. In case of fasting, the mother can lose some of the integral nutrients and the overall consequences can be destructive and complicated.

During pregnancy and even after pregnancy, all along nursing, women should not try the intermittent fasting because it could cause them and the baby some of the health challenges. However, they will put on some weight and, to keep themselves active and fatigue free, they need to try some physical workout, in order to avoid any muscle cramp or other issues.

In fact, after pregnancy and nursing, women could decide to undertake the intermittent fasting to help them to get back to shape and to avoid any health issue; even in this case they need to be conscious about what and when they are eating.

Different effects of intermittent fasting

Women can face different effects of intermittent fasting. It is not just limited to women, but every human being can face different reactions of fating in general. For females, their situation is a little tricky, due to the sudden hormonal changes or imbalances: there may be occur other changes in a female body that makes the body sensitive to calorie restriction.

Some of them may feel different in their hormonal cycle, while others face the change in menstrual cycle. Moreover, it can lead to the mood swings and cramps at times. Female's body is sensitive to changes, so in some cases a woman could suffer from cognition problems or low blood sugar. In this regard, the ultimate safe side is the selection of right meal plan: women need to ensure that they will choose an arrangement that suits their body type and hormonal level as well.

Important guidelines

For all women who want to get start with intermittent fasting they need to focus on the following guidelines:

- Consider your meal intake preferences
- Select a meal plan for intermittent fasting that suits your casual routine
- Do not shift to the intermittent fasting meal plan instantly
- Take the small intervals in the beginning and then increase your fasting span
- Make sure to have a test run of your selected meal plan to avoid issues
- Observe any of your hormonal changes, menstrual cycle changes or mood swings
- Do not try intermittent fasting if you want to conceive, to be pregnant or nursing a new born
- Always make sure to eat healthy in your meals to meet up the nutrient requirements in the body

Fasting And Diabetics

This diet is ideal to control diabetes; it is one of the popular and well-known benefits of the intermittent fasting. However, there is a fine line between the categories of diabetes. Commonly, people confuse the type of diabetes that can be treated with the help of intermittent fasting with the one that is incurable. There is no doubt that people can overcome their diabetes that is not supported by medicine; if a person is taking insulin and other diabetic medicines, then it is not possible to treat it completely with the intermittent fasting.

Know your type

If you are suffering from diabetes and you want to control it using the intermittent fasting, then make sure you are going to identify the diabetic type. Once you have the idea about the type, consequently you could decide whether intermittent fasting is for you or not. People who have issues with their blood sugar level and they are in a pre-diabetic stage, they may look for an appropriate solution in the intermittent fasting.

In case of severe diabetes where patient takes insulin to sustain sugar level, he/she should not do the intermittent fasting. In such conditions, the person can face critical issues such as:

- Low levels of blood sugar
- Unconsciousness
- Life threatening situations
- Loss of control and coordination
- Intolerance to meal plans
- Drop in blood pressure and more
- Make a careful selection

For all the diabetic patients it is necessary to make a careful selection with their meal plan and intermittent fasting. It is not impossible for them to try out the intermittent fasting, but they need to pick up a suitable strategy. They cannot opt for a regular strategy, but they can take one day or alternative strategies as well.

Bottom Line

It is not necessary that intermittent fasting is good enough for everyone. Everyone has specific body requirements and everyone should treat their body accordingly. In order to get the right and maximum benefits of a specific method it is important to use it right. For the kids and the elder who are unable to sustain without food, fasting is not an ideal option. Anyone who wants to control the body weight and mass should look for alternative approaches, instead of risking your own life.

Before starting up with the intermittent fasting, you always have the option to select the meal plan after trying it out. Make sure to gather the whole information about the meal plan and to select the right options for you, then you can make a real difference in the overall situation. In case of any problem with your fasting plan, you can always quit the plan and look for the medical help if needed.

Chapter 4
Intermittent Fasting With Keto Diet

When you are focusing on the intermittent fasting for weight loss, then you get to know about something else that is even magical. The keto diet follows the ketosis process to reduce the body fats and makes you lose weight. Combining both can simply trigger the results and get you the maximum benefits; if you want to have the quick results, then make sure that these are the best options for you. All you need is to incorporate both methods together and follow the plans keenly.

You can list out all the keto recipes for the meal times in your intermittent fasting, and you can take the keto meal, according to the plan. Doing so, you will get the double results from the both ends. On the one hand the intermittent fasting will help you to improve digestion and metabolism, on the other hand, keto diet will help to burn fats from the body and bring an amazing transformation.

Keto Diet & Its Health Benefits

Keto diet is a diet combination that comes with no carbs or fiber, but high fats in food. The meal plans in ketosis are based on all fats that increase the fat burning producer in the muscles. Eventually, it helps to lose weight and get lean muscles that consequently help to mark the ultimate body transformation.

Keto diet is not just a method to reduce weight but it comes with a combination of multiple benefits: just as if the intermittent fasting gives health benefits that are good enough to give you a healthy and well-balanced life style.

Weight reduction

One of the core outcomes of the keto diet is the weight reduction. Although it is a high, fats diet with no fiber and carbs, it burns body fats and let the person to be in good shape.

Healthy skin

This diet is not only effective for the weight loss and fat burning but also for healthy skin: it helps to increase the blood flow and make the skin looks attractive, radiant and beautiful.

Improve liver health

Commonly, we have issues with the blood purification that is due to poor functioning of liver. Keto diet helps the liver to work properly and reduces the fatty liver from the body; furthermore, it gives better quality of blood and its circulation in the body.

Reduced risk of diabetes type 2

The studies explain that, with the adoption of this diet, people suffering or diagnosed with type 2 diabetes got better coverage of blood sugar levels, because it helps them to control the blood sugar in their body that reduces the chances of critical condition and medications as well.

Improved heart health

Keto diet decreases the chances of cholesterol and health problems while on the other hand it increases heart life: the proper blood circulation and better arteries are the reason behind improved heart health.

Better brain functioning

If you have a well-planned keto diet plan, you will be able to improve the brain functioning. The more you will feel better and fresh, the better it will be for you to understand and to process the information.

Improved PCOS conditions

In women, PCOS is one of the common and problematic medical conditions, as it causes a number of factors such as infertility, change of hormones, obesity, and many others. With the help of ketogenic diet, women are able to control all the negative impacts of the PCOS. In fact, they can have the improved health situation that will help them to deal with the complications easily.

Do's & Don'ts In Keto Diet

Overall keto diet is generally safe for everyone but in exceptional cases, such as elders, kids, pregnant women and others, there is a need of consideration. Just like the other methods, it is necessary to make sure that you are not going to make any random decision about following keto diet and intermittent fasting together. There are certain do's and don'ts of the keto diet that you should know before jumping into it. These guidelines can help you make the best out of what you are going to do, so make sure to go through the guidelines keenly.

What you should do in keto diet?

There is something that comes favorable when you are following a keto diet and some things are acceptable. In your acceptable things, you will get the option to use a product but not in abundance. Here are some things that you can include in the meal plan:

Fats and proteins

In your keto meal plan, you need to have all the meal designs and adjusted in a high ratio or proteins and fats. The more fats you will have in the meal, the best it will be for you. Make sure you are going to pick up the animal fat and protein, instead of any artificial source of proteins.

Portion everything

It is ideal to have the portion of multiple things in your plate. As you cannot get much rice and bread, you need to add on some portions to the food in order to will help you to get the belly filled.

Provide yourself variations

Meat, eggs and cheese can be boring for you in a long run. You need to find out some other variations for your meal plan, so it is necessary for you to evaluate what can be the different on the menu. There are a lot of keto recipes out there, so you can pick up any of these attractive and interesting recipes. These will help you to make a real difference in your overall diet routine.

Plan all the meals in detail

The time for keto diet plan varies from a person to person: there is not any boundary for the time that you will get results in a specific standard. Things can be different for you and to others as well. As a matter of fact, all you need to do is to design the plan for first 3 months initially; this will help you to identify how your body reacts to it. Later on, you can continue the plan for further time.

Make sure to plan all the meals separately. It includes that you will have a whole schedule for different breakfast, lunch or dinner options with you. It will help you to stick to the diet and have better results. On the other hand, multiple options in food will help you to get the different kinds of nutrients.

Use of dairy products

Using the abundance of all dairy products is not an ideal option in keto diet. You may find the use of cheese and butter in abundance in all the keto recipes, due to high fats. Differently, you need to take only Greek yoghurt as a snack; the limit for the yoghurt is one cup or one and a half cup, not more than that.

Things to avoid in keto diet

Just like any other diet plan, keto diet comes with some limitations and restrictions. Ketosis is a chemical procedure that happens to your body due to the high protein and fat food you take in routine. If you are not taking the food as per guided pattern, then you will not be able to hit the right results. Here are some things you need to avoid when following a keto diet plan:

No alcohol

The use of alcohol could cause you trouble with the keto diet, as it can put effect on your stomach and eventually reduces your psychological hold. Any imbalance with the brain can cause your body to react differently and the stomach can lead to adverse reactions.

Avoid sugar

Any sugar item, especially the artificial sugar, is one of the restrictions in the keto diet plan. Sugar intake increases your blood sugar level instantly and it is not a good sign, as you will not be able to consume the energy and it will not help you to reduce weight. Furthermore, you need to quit all the sweet food other than the natural sweets like fruits.

Limit the carbs

Keto diet is a no carb diet. You need to avoid everything that contains carbs; it is a kind of hard thing to do and it causes you keto flu as well, because our body is not good enough sometimes to adjust. However, with a little try, you can get used to it and things will be in your favor.

Avoid starch in abundance

In your keto meal plans, there is not space for the starch food products like potato, sweet potato, rice and more. It is not a hard and fat rule to cut off these products, but limit them to use; you can avoid the maximum use and occasionally incorporate these options in your diet.

Keto Diet With Intermittent Fasting & Weight Loss

It seems to be a perfect combination if you plan to mix up the intermittent fasting with keto diet meal plans. It is not a difficult issue, as it will give you some quick results. At one side, you will have a fat cutting diet plan that will help you to reduce the body fats naturally by melting them off. On the other hand, the fasting period will help you so that the keto diet works efficiently. It is one of a system that can work for you in a long run. You can pick up the combination for quick and long-term results. Moreover, both methods do have their own benefits, so you will be able to get both of these in one package.

Some points to consider:

If you have plans to start keto meal and intermittent fasting together, then you need to focus on the following points:

- Plan your diet according to your exertion and regular meal requirements
- Select a moderate fasting plan in the beginning and then take it to the next level
- Always have a trial for both in separate or combination and then make your final call
- Do not repeat the same meals but incorporate some new things to excite your taste buds
- In case of any side effect or reaction of the routine, make sure to take an exit
- You need to practice things initially and then go smoothly with everything ahead

Chapter 5
Metabolic Autophagy

The word autophagy is derived from two Greek words "auto" and "phagein"; these two words mean "self" and "eating".

It is a body mechanism to break down all the machinery of old cells. In the list of these old cells proteins, organelles, and cell membranes are included. When you have no energy in your body because of less eating, this mechanism helps you to have sustain energy by regulating the cells, by recycling and deteriorating the components of cells.

You fast for a short time and eat healthy food in autophagy. Healthy food contains low carbs and high fats. It is a simple and easy way to lose weight and gain health benefits.

How Does Autophagy Work?

It works be keeping in the maintenance mode. It perfectly activates in the situation of stress, and its objective is to protect your body, helping you to slow down your aging process. It boosts the natural ability to perform your body's functions. It also reduces the chances of different diseases by reducing inflammation.

Intermittent fasting:

While doing autophagy it is better to do intermittent fasting; you should choose the 16:8 fasting, which is the best option. With this option, you fast for 16 hours and eat in the remaining 8 hours; be careful, you cannot ignore its importance in losing weight and keeping you fit.

Metabolic autophagy:

Your body's metabolism has two sub-sections or categories: the first is anabolism and the second is catabolism. Anabolism is used to build in your body new physical matters, while the catabolism is used to break down the molecules. Thanks to this, you get the energy that helps in the digestion of food.

Therefore, metabolic autophagy means to maintain a balance between anabolism and catabolism, as it has an effective impact on your body and it expands your lifespan as well. By combining these two, this method helps to replaced or construct all the damaged portions of cells by bringing back the cells after constructing them in the energy steam.

With this, in real words, your body eats itself. On the other hand, it helps you to maintain homeostasis.

Benefits of autophagy

Autophagy is a process that cleans your body's damaged cells and harmful toxins and it supports you to generate new and healthy cells. Furthermore, it also trains your body to eat itself.

It became really popular because of its advantages, apart from losing weight, it has other positive impacts too that keep your life healthy.

The most salient features or benefits of autophagy are discussed here.

Metabolism works better:

Autophagy's major feature is to keep your cells healthy, by replacing all the damaged cells parts and throwing away all the toxics, as your body cells help to burn your body fats. If they work properly, they will keep you healthy and fit, because it repairs or replaces the most important part of the cell, which is called mitochondria.

Mitochondria is a part of a cell that actually burns your body fat. Besides burning your body fat, it makes the ATP, which is the energetic currency of your body. Along with the other things your cells also have some toxics that build up in the cells and damaged them badly, but getting rid of these toxins you can save your cells from harm. Moreover, it helps your cell function in more appropriate and efficient way; with this, not only your body fat burns but it also helps to make protein. All these features help your metabolism works better.

Weight loss:

For weight loss, the process is an amazing element. Besides getting other health benefits weight loss comes at the top of the list. Through this, your body fats burn without damaging the protein. Autophagy activates in the short fasts burning them and preserving muscle mass and proteins.

Besides that, it also reduces the insulin levels in the body, which helps to lessen the inflammation and it stops you to gain weight. Furthermore, it also helps the cells by repairing it and it assisting in burning the fats to get energy.

Save your life:

Autophagy is an old mechanism that plays a vital role in preserving your life. Firstly, it works effectively when your body is stressed, starved, or infected. During these hard times, autophagy comes into action by minimizing the damage and by doing maximum repair.

With the combination of intermittent fasting, autophagy's function gives better results: both of these starve your body's glucose contagious intruder, as it helps to boost your immune system by reducing inflammation. Animals use this technique to preserve their energy and to repair their damaged cells.

In the case of the human body, its immune system is critical; however, with autophagy, your immune system fights illnesses and reduces the risks of various illnesses. All its functions have a huge impact on your overall health and it saves your life by healing and replacing the dead cells with healthy cells.

Maintain homeostasis:

Because of this, you get a vibrant health. It helps you to maintain your homeostasis. Homeostasis is a function that balances your body cells, due to this function, your body's dead cells are removed and it forms new cells.

Improve your quality of life:

When we talk about anti-aging term it is not only related to your skin beauty. Anti-aging is a deeper term that goes deeper from your skin. Autophagy is an ancient method and scientists have known about this since 1950s.

280

However, in the past it was not common but now, because of its advantages, various studies have been conducted on this process.

The last researches have shown that it is perfect for improving your cellular health by repairing them. This process does not replace the whole cell but it repairs the damaged part of the it; besides that, it also removes all the toxic elements and fixes the cells.

After the process of repairing, your cells start to work in a better and efficient way, by working like new and younger cells. You will notice that some people look younger from their actual age. On the other hand, few people seem older than their actual age and the reason behind these two conditions is the efficiency and condition of the cells. If your body has toxic and damaged cells, it will affect you in a negative way, and you will look older than your biological age. Moreover, if your damaged cells are repaired on time, it will keep you look young and fresh, so these cells play a crucial role in your appearance.

Improves brain health:

Indeed, autophagy plays a vital role in improving your brain health. In many people, brain diseases develop at a later age, and the reason behind these brain diseases is the misfolded protein around and in the brain. Autophagy removes the misfolded or useless protein that automatically prevents you from different brain diseases; for instance, the disease like Parkinson and Alzheimer can be prevented or delayed.

Regulate inflammation:

Regulation of inflammation is very important to save yourself from diseases because it boosts your immune system and helps you to combat diseases; furthermore, it addresses the issues that trigger the inflammation and by controlling them, it reduces the rate of inflammation.

Improve digestive system:

We all know that the digestive system plays a crucial role in your life. Your life depends on your digestive system, that means: if the liver works properly, only then your body will get essential substances. The process of Autophagy helps you to improve your digestive function by removing and replacing the damaged cells, and it finally enhances the function of liver. Lastly, with the fast, your liver gets a break to reschedule its function.

The process also removes all the junk that is based on unhealthy and useless toxics or cells. By activating autophagy with a perfect schedule, it will help you. Try to expand your fast to overnight, as with this, your digestive system will get the time to heal itself.

Protects from infectious diseases:

As autophagy strengthens your immune system, it protects you from infectious diseases, by giving you the strength to fight against them. Moreover, it eliminates certain microbes from the cell, such as HIV, Mycobacterium tuberculosis; besides, it does not only removes directly the cell part but it also removes the toxins that are created by the infections.

Improves muscle performance:

You can improve your muscle's performance through this process. After exercise, your muscles need repair and they want energy too. Through autophagy your muscle cells will react immediately, it will improve the energy balance and will reduce the risk of damage in future.

Minimize the apoptosis:

Autophagy plays an important role in dealing with apoptosis. This process is dangerous for cells as it caused the cell's death. Your body generates some inflammation to clean the mess of dead cells, but it is not enough. In this situation, autophagy steps forward by selecting the cells that can't be repaired and by dumping them.

Prevent cancer:

It also lowers the inflammation and reduces the chronic inflammations that can cause cancer. As we see, various types of cancers are increasing rapidly. One of the common cancers is breast cancer.

You will be amazed to know that with autophagy the chances of cancer reduce, as it responds quickly against chronic inflammation, DNA damage response, and genome instability; it also suppresses the process of cancer development.

Improves your skin health:

To look beautiful, you must have good skin. You cannot get good skin by using moisturizers and other beauty products, your skin beauty also relates to your diet. An appropriate diet provides your skin nutrients.

You damage your skin cells by working in the daylight and by exposing to dust; furthermore, skin cells also are mostly affected by bacteria. Through autophagy, you can a glowing and clear skin, it also removes the damaged cells and last, but not least, it repairs the cells and removes the bacteria from the skin.

Diet Should Follow Autophagy:

Diet plays an important role in achieving your goals through autophagy. You must be careful about what you are eating: the first and most essential feature is to low your carbohydrates and calories intake and secondly, increase your protein intake.

Low-carbs food:

The reason behind lowering the carbs in your diet is to use your body fats. Yes, your body will force to use its fats as a source of fuel. With low carbs you need to take food with high fats because proteins can turn into the carb, whereas the situation is different in the fats.

Protein consumption:

You need to limit your proteins once or twice a week. Restrict protein limit to 15-25 grams. With this, your body gets the time to recycle its proteins. It reduces the inflammation and cleanses your cells; while cleaning your cells, it does not cause muscle loss. Whilst you are not taking the proteins, your body uses the proteins by consuming its toxins.

Diet is compulsory:

During autophagy diet is compulsory, as you will not be able to achieve your goals without following a proper diet plan. Set the time for eating and fasting and during the eating hours don't try to eat any unhealthy food, is prohibited during autophagy.

Metabolic Disorders & Autophagy

Metabolic disorders are affecting human life in a negative way, due to the change of lifestyle and environmental aspects. Besides, the main threat is the metabolic disorders. Autophagy is considered the best solution to avoid metabolic disorders. Indeed, various recent studies are showing the positive effects of autophagy on human life.

What are the metabolic disorders?

Metabolism is an important function of your body so that it uses this chemical process to transform the food you have eaten into the fuel or energy, and this energy keeps you alive.

When your body's metabolism process fails, then metabolic disorders emerged. Due to its failure, your body either gets less or gets much of the essential substances, and both situations are harmful to your health.

Our bodies are sensitive and cannot tolerate the error of metabolism. When your liver stops to function in a proper way, metabolic disorders occurred.

Common metabolic disorders:

Metabolic disorders are complex and cause various complications. These are life taking disorders.

Diabetes:

The most common metabolic disorder is diabetes and, unfortunately, the number of patients with diabetes is increasing rapidly.

Gaucher's disease:

This disease occurred when a specific kind of fat doesn't break down due to the liver's inappropriate functioning.

Hereditary hemochromatosis:

It is a condition that emerged with an excessive amount of iron in different body organs. With this metabolic disorder a man can lose his life, as it can cause liver cancer, heart disease, diabetes, and liver cirrhosis.

What is autophagy?

According to the physiology, autophagy is known as a protective housekeeping mechanism. With its mechanism, it eliminates all the unhealthy cells and toxins. In its cellular function it aggregates the protein, constructs the damaged organelles, and invades pathogen through a dependent pathway of lysosome.

Obesity:

Obesity is the most serious concern and a threat to a large number of populations. Due to the eating disorders and unhealthy eating people are becoming the victim of obesity. Obesity is also causing various other diseases, such as diabetes, heart diseases, and so on.

Relationship between metabolic disorders and autophagy:

Autophagy is protecting you from these metabolic illnesses, for instance, in obesity, autophagy plays the role of an internal source as it provides the stored nutrients during the limitation of nutrients.

As metabolic disorders can take your life you need to take preventive measures. In a few cases, there is no cure and a person can die within months, and the cause behind the metabolic disorders is the imbalance distribution of essential substances.

At this stage, the autophagy comes into action: it recycles the macromolecules and regulates the cellular homeostasis; furthermore, it cleans the damaged organelles and proteins. Recent studies showed that autophagy plays an important role in improving the human life, by preventing a person from all these metabolic disorders, or by decreasing the risks of metabolic disorders.

It repairs the cells of all the body organs and removes all the toxic and dead cells. This function enhances the function of the organs. The liver works in an effective way and it also helps with obesity and insulin resistance.

Moreover, it also eliminates all the useless amounts of the essential substance. So, it helps in balancing the cells and their functions; moreover it automatically decreases the chances of metabolic disorders.

Chapter 6
Intermittent Fasting 101 Methods

Here is a complete guide about the Intermittent fasting methods that are available and you can use to make a difference. These are not something unusual, but they are recommended and used methods that actually work. Commonly, people think that intermittent fasting is a kind of starving that appears to be a torture for people. In fact, it is not like that: intermittent fasting is a systematic management of the calories, food intake and its consumption as well.

Everyone has multiple options for the intermittent fasting methods. All these methods are effective and give results. Moreover, these methods make the fasting save for everyone. If you follow the right methods for the intermittent fasting, you will not starve your body; in fact, you will be providing all the necessary nutrients in the right timings.

The best thing about these methods is the management of your whole day and meal. It is not just the time but also the calorie management, so you can have the idea about what to eat and what not. You can opt the things that will help you to make a difference in the overall scenario, so make sure to select these methods carefully that are near to your potential and stamina. This will help you to get the right results from the intermittent fasting practice in a long run.

Advantages Of Intermittent Fasting:

Intermittent fasting is really good for your health because it helps you not only in losing weight but also it looks after your health. The top benefits and positive effects of intermittent fasting are discussed here.

Lose weight:

The basic reason behind intermittent fasting is losing weight; it is an effective way to lose weight, because you eat less and healthy. Moreover, it enhances your hormone's function and helps to reduce weight. With this your body fats burnt and you achieve your goal in a limited time.

Physical fitness:

Besides preventing neurodegenerative disorders, it also helps you to remain fit. With intermittent fasting your metabolism works efficiently, by training your digestive system and by taking care of that you will eat in a limited time frame; it also trains you to eat only when you feel hungry. Moreover, you started to eat healthy food.

Some people believe that fasting damage your metabolism. It is totally a wrong perception. If you fast and eat in a proper way, it helps your metabolism by making it better, using fats and glucose efficiently for energy.

Expand your life span:

It expands your life span by improving the liver function, as you are giving a rest to your liver, and by fasting, its lifespan is extended. So, your liver becomes healthier and functions effectively.

Prevents from Alzheimer's disease:

As we all know, Alzheimer is a neurodegenerative disorder and it is not a curable disease; therefore, it is important to take preventive measures. A study shows that intermittent fasting reduces the chances of Alzheimer because it plays a positive role in reducing its complications by improving the symptoms.

It is also acclaimed that intermittent fasting protects from other neurodegenerative diseases too, such as Huntington and Parkinson.

16:8 Fasting Method

It is an easy, effective and most popular way of intermittent fasting. It is a sustained and convenient weight loss technique that also improves your health. 16:8 fasting method allows you to restrict eating time to 8 to 10 hours a day. In this method you fast for 16 hours every day and during the 8 hours of eating you can take 2 to 3 meals.

It is a simple method and you can easily do it. So, you are just skipping your breakfast. If you finish your dinner at 8 pm and do not eat anything till 12 pm the next day, you completed your fast; it means that you have just skipped your breakfast and have completed your 16 hours fast. For women, though, it is recommended to do fast for

14 to 15 hours, because for them 16 hours fasting is too much time.

You can set the cycle of 16:8 fasting; this totally depends on your preferences. So, you can do it on a regular basis, which means every day. Moreover, you can also do this twice or thrice a week. There are not any hard and fast rules like other dieting fasts, it is a flexible diet plan that can easily fit in your daily routine.

Health benefits of 16:8 fasting:

The most important benefit of 16:8 fasting is that it attacks obesity. Yes, you can lose weight and save yourself from all the diseases related to obesity. Besides losing weight, you can also enjoy a bunch of health benefits, for example, it reduces the chances of heart diseases, cancer, inflammation, cholesterol level, and blood sugar levels, it is very effective for your mental health as well.

Is it right for me?

The first question that raised in a person's mind is: is it right for me? The answer to this question is yes, 16:8 fasting is right for you. Because of this you lose your weight and it also has a positive impact on your overall health.

One thing that you should keep in mind is eating healthy food. The food must be nutritious and organic so, there is no room for processed food or food with artificial sugar. If you will not eat nutritious food, fasting will not help you at all.

Recommendations:

If you have any health issues it is better to consult your doctor before fasting. For example, if you are diabetic, or have other issues, this can put you in trouble. For children, underweight individuals, pregnant girls, it is not a good choice. So, if you have any problems, don't fast without an expert's consultation because you can face serious consequences.

What Is 20:4?

20:4 is one of the types of intermittent fasting where you fast for 20 hours and you can eat during the 4 hours. It is slightly different from warrior diet, as in this you cannot eat anything during the 20 hours of the day, while in the 4 hours you can have a big meal. It is a very common type of intermittent fasting.

It is a bit strict fasting as compared to others. In 20:4, unlike the warrior diet, you have to stick with the ketogenic diet. Yes, in warrior diet you just stuck to the low calorie's food, but in this you are supposed to eat limited items even in eating hours. You can set the eating time and fasting time according to your comfort.

What to eat after completing the 20:4 fast?

You need to eat healthy, nutritious and ketogenic food, and it is best to start eating gradually. Unlike warrior diet, try to start eating from snacks, then gradually keep eating small portion of meals in the 4 hour-time duration. Some people eat a proper meal right after finishing the fast, and then eat snacks in the remaining time of 4 hours. The second method is okay too, but it is recommended to start with snacks.

You can eat white fish, green leafy vegetables, water, dark coffee, broth, and low carb vegetables.

What happens during 20:4 fast?

You are not eating anything for 20 hours, but you are eating only ketogenic food in the 4 hours eating time period. This diet will put pressure on your body to use its glycogen stores that is the storage part of carbohydrates. In its reaction, your body will start burning your body fats and if you do not eat for long hours, it will lower the stay of insulin levels, so your liver will mobilize and start to use your body fats as a fuel.

Long Fasts

Shorter time duration fast is common and is in trend. People fast for short hours to lose weight, but besides short hour fasts, you can go for a long fast, like 5:2, 16:8, 20:4 are the short duration fasts. In the list of long fasts, 24 hours, 36 hours and 48 hours fasts come. The longest intermittent fast is of a duration of 48 hours.

What to drink during long hours fast?

In a long hour fasting you give yourself and your liver a full one or more than one-day break. During these two days you don't eat anything but you can drink fluids with zero-calories. You can drink water, tea, and black coffee; water is an essential fluid and if you do not drink water, your body will be dehydrated. So, drink plenty of water to keep your body hydrated during long fasts.

What to eat after completing a long fast?

In shorter fasts, you can eat any healthy food in big portion; however, after completing the longest fast of intermittent fasting, you can't eat in big portion, so you need to start eating in small portions and gradually. Start your meal from light snacks and take a small portion of meal after two hours.

If you start eating instantly, it will put you in trouble because it can cause diarrhea or nausea.

How many times you can have a long fast in a month?

Long hour fasts are not an easy task. Everyone cannot do this. You cannot have long fasts twice or once a week, it is strictly prohibited. So, it is suggested to have a long fast one or twice a month. As if you do it with short breaks, it can affect your health in negative way.

Benefits of long fast on health:

Long fast have positive effects on your health. You put an effort and it paid off. With long fast, you find the best results: your body fats burn at a great speed and it not only helps you to lose weight, it also helps you to maintain your health.

It also plays an important role in preventing neurological disorders because it reduces the risks of cardiovascular diseases and few cancers. Moreover, it expands your lifespan and it gives you a healthy lifespan as well. Lastly, it improves your metabolism and combat inflammation that can cause various diseases.

Fast Diet – 5:2

The fast diet 5:2 is also called the 5:2 diet. It has a symbolic name that means eating 5 days normally and limiting calories on the remaining 2 days. Here fast is a misleading term, like another intermittent fasting, you don't restrict yourself from eating for a certain time because you just limit your calorie intake. On fasting days, you just intake around 25 percent calories, as compared to normal days.

This diet was introduced by a British doctor and journalist named Michael Mosley. It is an easy effective dieting method of intermittent fasting; it does not require 16 hours fasting nor 10-hour fasting. You normally eat 5 days a week and in this method you just need to sacrifice your 2 days. Yes, only 2 days a week. You restrict yourself to 500 to 600 calories on two days of a week.

What to eat on a fast day?

In fast diet-5:2 you can eat at any time but you need to be careful about what you are eating, because you are supposed to eat food that is rich in nutrients and it must have all the basic elements like protein and fiber.

Vegetables:

If you start fast diet-5:2, then eat more vegetables, as it will give you a satisfaction of tummy-filling. Vegetables have low calories, so you can take more vegetables at a time, eating carrots, zucchini, and green leafy vegetables; all these vegetables are healthy and provide you enough amount of fiber.

Eggs and whitefish:

Protein is vital while you are fasting or not, so you should eat the food with protein but with less fat. Therefore, you can take hard-boiled egg, white fish, tofu, beans, lentils, peas, and cuts of lean animal. You can use these items after boiling, roasting, or grilling; don't fry them, as it will add fats in it.

Other food items:

Along with vegetables and protein food, you have some other options too, such as drinking water a lot. Fast days doesn't stop you from drinking water as water is vital. You can also eat fruits with less sugar, blueberries, and blackberries, for instance; soup or broth are also effective in intake during fast day.

Patterns of eating:

You get a room while fasting 5:2. It doesn't restrict you from eating for long hours, so you can eat at any time of the day. For helping you the 2 most effective eating pattern is described here: one is three small meals and second is two slightly bigger meals.

Three small meals:

In this eating pattern, you take a meal 3 times a day. You do breakfast, lunch, and dinner, but all these meals are small in quantity.

Two slightly bigger meals:

You eat twice a day in this eating pattern. You skip one meal and eat medium-sized meals twice a day.

During both, the patterns must focus on nutritious food. The food must be low in calories and fats, it must be rich in protein and fiber too, and don't cross your limit of calories.

24 & 36 Hours Fasting

Intermittent fasting has different types of fasts that differ in duration too. 24 and 36-hour fasting are also 2 types of intermittent fasting. You can opt any one type of fasting, depending on your feasibility.

What is 24-hour fasting?

24-hour fasting, as the name suggested, is a fast of 24 hours. From your last dinner to the next day's dinner you can set the time according to your comfort; it is an effective method of losing weight, as it covers more hours with fasting, in order to get the results soon. You are eating at least one meal a day.

For losing weight it is recommended to do thrice a week. For some people it is easy to fast for 24 hours. Therefore, to get the results soon they fast 5 times a week.

What is 36-hour fasting?

It is a total fast of 36 long hours where you don't eat anything for consecutive 36 hours. It is an amazing way to reduce weight for even diabetic patients. Doctors recommended diabetic patients to have a 36 hour fast twice or thrice a week. With 36 hours fasting you get quicker results.

Disclaimer:

Fasting for 24 or 36 hours is not equally benefited for everyone. For some people, such as underweight people, ladies who are pregnant or doing breastfeeding, boys or girls under the age of 18, it is not beneficial and not recommended to fast. In addition to this, people who have eating disorders or any health challenges should not fast for 24 hours or 36 hours.

If you want to fast, then it is suggested to try it with short time duration fast. It is ideal to start fasting from 5:2 or from 16:8 fasting; if you complete those fasts, then do 24 and 36-hour fasting.

Fasting In Alternative Days

As its name suggested, fasting in alternative days means that you fast every other day. You will find its various versions. Some believe that you need to restrict yourself to around 500 calories during a fast day, but on the non-fasting days you are allowed to eat anything; it is an effective weight-loss method. While fasting you can drink calorie-free drinks, like water, tea, and black coffee.

An easier way to lose weight:

This fasting is also known as "every other day diet". People find it much easier as a way to lose weight, as they can stick to this comfortably, and also because you restrict your calories, rather than remain hungry for a long time. With this fasting you get the same results as you get from the other long hour fasts.

A study's results showed that fasting alternative days have various positive effects: you preserve muscle mass along with burning your body fats quickly, and if you start exercise along with the fasting alternative days, it will be a cherry on the top, because you will start to lose weight at double speed.

Is it safe to do fasting in alternative days?

Studies have shown that fasting in alternative days is safer than others. It suits most of the people. One of the major benefits that you get from this fasting is amazing, as long as you don't gain the weight again. In those methods, the week you stop fasting, you start to see the changes in weight. It also decreases anxiety, depression and overeating.

Impulsive Fasting

Most of the body changes we observe in ourselves are due to impulsive or mindless eating. When we are sad, we eat, when we are happy, we eat, we use to have dinners, brunches and lunches to celebrate anything. In short, for everything, we have only one way out and that is eating. Eventually, it gives us a huge feedback in the form of massive weight gain and a bad shape body as well. To fix up the problem it is important to treat it the way it needs to be.

Intermittent fasting brings you the option of impulsive fasting that brings you the pattern of fasting, similar to our food intake. As we do not think for once at least to eat anything, same as this is one of the random and rash fasting types. You adopt fasting randomly to make sure you will starve enough to let your body consume stored energy.

Not a harsh game

Many people think that impulsive fasting is harsh one. They believe that you are torturing yourself by keeping the body starve for food in different timings. In real, it is about building your capacity to control food cravings and manage the overall metabolism. No matter it is an impulsive form of fasting, but still you need to consider the diet schedule.

A careful selection

The most important thing with the impulsive fasting is the selection of schedule. Although there is no specific schedule for the fasting, you need to make careful selection. Fasting does not refer you to risk your life. So, make sure you are going to take the meals at appropriate time. You need to keep the fast long enough that you can handle easily.

Not a fixed fasting chart

It is not necessary that you need to follow a fixed fasting chart in the impulsive fasting. If one day you have a meal in the morning and then after the 8 hours break, you will take another meal; then, on the second day, you may take the first meal in the afternoon. The timings are different and random, so your body will get the different treatment every time.

Warrior Fasting

Warrior fasting was first introduced by Ori Hofmekler, who is a famous author in the field of health and fitness. He proposed this fasting in 2001, after observing its effects on himself and his friends in the Israeli special force. With this fasting, you can lose your weight in short time span.

Warrior fasting is actually based on the ancient warriors eating patterns. They used to eat less during the day and eat a lot at dinner. Hofmekler described this fasting as "it is designed to improve the way we eat, feel, perform and look".

Warrior fasting involves fasting for 20 long hours. These 20 hours include night and day time. After 20 hours you do over eating in the 4 hours duration. These 4 hours must be the evening hours.

Not a scientific study:

Warrior fasting weight loss strategy is not a scientific study, but it is based on a person's observation. Thus, there is no research-based answers that are available on its effectiveness. Even Hofmekler also said that he didn't propose it after experiment; it is totally based on his observations. He observed this during his stay in the military force, so that's why he named it warrior fasting or warrior diet.

What to eat?

There is no specific food to eat in warrior fasting, so you can take any food with healthy fats and protein. If the food is organic and nutritious you can take it. However, it is prohibited to take food that is processed or has artificial sugar.

The most common food items that you can take during the 4 hours eating break are listed here.

- Hard-boiled eggs
- Dairy products like milk, cottage cheese, yoghurt
- Grains like rice, bread, oatmeal, and so on
- Chicken or beef broth
- Fruits like mango, banana, apples, pineapples, strawberries, peach, kiwi, grapes, pomegranate, and so on
- Raw vegetables for example peas, green leafy vegetables, carrots, mushrooms, onion, and so on
- Vegetal juices of carrot, beet, celery, and so on.

Benefits of Warrior fasting:

Warrior fasting is gaining the attention of the dietitians because of its results. Consequently, it has various benefits that help you a lot in different dimensions. A few major advantages of warrior fasting are discussed here.

Weight loss:

Fasting, as we all know, has a history and helps a lot in weight loss. Warrior diet is also one of the intermittent fasting types that helps you to lose weight in small duration because of 20 hours fasting you lose a certain amount of your body fats. With this you not only lose weight, but the chances of cardiovascular disease are also minimized.

Inflammation:

Inflammation is the leading cause of major diseases. For example, few types of cancers, heart diseases, bowel disorder, diabetes, and many others. Warrior fasting helps to fight against chronic inflammation.

Improve blood sugar:

Like other fasting methods, with warrior fasting, you will see improvement in your blood sugar, as it controls your blood sugar and insulin. However, it will only happen when you eat the right food during eating hours.

Side effects of warrior fasting:

Besides its advantages, it has many side effects too, for example, it is not an ideal weight-loss method for everyone. Some of the major side effects of warrior fasting are given below.

- Lightheadedness
- Dizziness
- Low energy
- Eating disorder
- Low blood sugar

- Hormonal imbalance
- Fainting
- Anxiety and depression
- Constipation

Protein Sparing Modified Fasting (PSMF)

Protein sparing modified fasting, which is also known as PSMF, is a way to lose weight. This method of weight loss was launched in 1970s. and the purpose of PSMF was to help people with obesity. In the past physicians used this method, but now, due to its effective and promising results, dietitians are also using it.

What is PSMF?

The PSMF is a diet containing low-calories and most protein. It is a weight-loss method that helps you to lose weight rapidly; in other words, "it is a diet with the goal to maintain muscle mass while losing body fats".

It is not an easy diet plan. However, it gives you great results in a short time period, as long as you take low-carbs and fats but it takes enough proteins that will preserve your lean tissue mass. Due to enough amount of protein, there are fewer chances of nutrient deficiencies.

Phases of PSMF:

A PSMF has two phases: the first is "intensive phase" and second is "refeeding phase".

Intensive phase:

The intensive phase of PSMF lasts for around 4-6 months. In this phase your diet contains fewer calories. The calories limit is less than 800 per day. Food like egg whites, fish, or chicken are lean protein foods but also have calories. Therefore, while eating something, you need to know what nutrition it has in store.

During this diet, you are allowed to take per day only 20-50 grams of carbohydrates. In simple words, you can take only 2 slices of bread. Considering protein intake, it varies person to person, because you need to take protein according to your body weight, like 1.2 to 1.5grams of protein per kilogram weight.

Fats are not allowed at all in the form of oils or dressings, because you are taking enough of your food.

Refeeding phase:

The refeeding phase lasts for around 6-8 weeks. In this phase, you start to gradually increase the calories intake back to normal levels. In this, the level of carbs increased to 45 grams in the first month, while in the second month, it raised up to 90grams.

There is no certain or underline limit of calories in this phase, because it will increase naturally by the addition of fats and carbs in the diet. Food that is high in protein and fiber will become a part of your diet, so you can take any fruit or vegetable that has low-fat in this phase.

Is it a safe method to lose weight?

It is very safe if you do it for a short time period and your goal is to just get a kick to start losing the weight. However, if you do it for the long-term, then you need to take some measures. For example, it is better to do it under medical supervision, because in long-duration you need to monitor various things, such as your gallstone, blood sugar levels, uric acid, and other features.

Although now we have a modified form of PSMF, it is different from the 1970s diet. Now it is more balanced and designed after research. In addition, it is suggested to do it under proper supervision.

Bottom Line

The multiple kinds of intermittent fasting allow you to have the ultimate access to the wonderful body transformation and weight loss. It is not a random technique to be good with your health but one of the refined methods that are used anciently. Although you have so many options in intermittent fasting, you need to pick any one of these carefully, as these are similar and interlinked and mixing up the random things can cause issues or problems later.

Chapter 7
How To Start With Intermittent Fasting?

"Skipping breakfast is not a healthier activity, having morning meal is an essential part of the day"
Unknown

Intermittent fasting is getting popular among people and almost everybody is talking about this. Is this becoming a way to lose weight? To have a healthier life? Or people do it for a religious purpose?

In general, intermittent fasting is the best practice to follow a healthy and fit life for a long time. According to several researches and studies, it is noticed that the proper and restrict way to have meals with a proper schedule, not only improves metabolism, but also gives multiple other benefits as well.

Before starting the intermittent fasting it is important to know that, what it is all about?

Intermittent fasting is basically a schedule and a way to have your meals in a day. During the fasting you have to follow a pattern in which your meals are divided according to the quantity and calories necessary to take in a day, in an hour respectively. There are multiple approaches regarding the intermittent fasting meal plans and people follow the one that suits them or fulfills their requirement.

How To Start Intermittent Fasting?

Choose the method

First of all, before starting, it is necessary to identify the method that a person is going to follow throughout the fasting process. There are multiple approaches or methods usually adopted by the people during the period like:

- Sometimes people may choose the eight-hour-method where they have food or meals and rest of sixteen hours do the fasting, and in the whole fasting, is only allowed to have a non-carbonated drinks and low calorie liquid intake like water, green tea, black tea or coffee without milk and sugar.
- Some people do the fasting in alternative days like having a restricted calorie diet in a week and fast for one day or two days a week.

Find out effects & probabilities

When you have selected one method of fasting, then do a proper research before applying it. In other words, it is vital to consult the health consultant or nutritionist because the expert can evaluate your body type and could suggest you the best and suitable method for you. Fasting directly could affect the metabolism of a person and may do some chemical changes that could have different consequences, according to the person. Anyway, all methods are suitable an appropriate for everyone. If you put your body in an intense method, perhaps the consequences can affect you badly.

Know what happen to body with fasting

With intermittent fasting the consequences are hormonal changes that take place inside the body. With the limited supply of the food and calories your body functions take place accordingly.

Fasting improve the production of hormones that are good for the muscle's growth and strength and it also helps to increase the utilization of energy that attains from the stored body fats. This will also keep the insulin level at the minimal rate, that means the body uses more stored body fats that put the body in the process of weight loss, so the body can fight more efficiently with the damage or dead cells and, finally, the body's ability to fight against disease goes high. Fasting is ultimately good for almost everyone, as well as it is an effective way to control over the weight and to follow the healthier lifestyle.

Benefits Of Following The Fasting

In general, people only think that maybe the fasting is just a way to lose weight or to fight against obesity; however, this is not the only reason to adopt the fasting because it has multiple other health benefits that helps people in multiple way who are following fasting. It includes:

Most importantly, we know that the intermittent fasting has a vital contribution in weight loss. According to the research it is showed up that people who are following the intermittent fasting follow the weight loss more rapidly than those who are not. Thus, it is an effective and quick way to lose weight and control over the calories than any other dieting method.

With intermittent fasting the metabolism function increased and helps with multiple health benefits, such as the reduction of the risk of heart disease, the decrease of the chances of diabetes and the control the blood inflammation Eventually, it is also helpful for obese people.

With good health and fitness, a person can live a long and healthy life. Besides, there is slow process of aging and a reduction of damaging the cell.

Most importantly, according to the health consultants and nutritionist, intermittent fasting is a safe an appropriate way to not only lose weight but also to improve the health. It is a completely new and organized way to have the meals that not only nourished the person health, but also gives a proper diet plans and charts to boost the overall body function.

Things To Consider Before Starting

No doubt, intermittent fasting is the best and result oriented way to not only reduce the weight but also improve the overall health condition. Moreover, it is important to know that before fasting, it is not appropriate for everyone, especially for people having some medical issues. Here are some people who cannot do the intermittent fasting, includes:

- Those who are under weight and do not have a healthier maintained body weight.
- If you have a digestive issue or a long history of some eating problem.
- The patients who are suffering from the chronical disease like high blood pressure, heart problem or diabetics. They are not allowed to put themselves on the intermittent fasting. If at any situation they have to do it, then they have to follow a doctor recommendation.
- Women who are pregnant and breastfeeding, are not allowed to follow the intermittent fasting.

That's all because the low calorie or strict diet ratio may be dangerous for such people and could cause different health complications.

Following the intermittent fasting is the challenging task for especially those who want to lose weight by restricting themselves with minimum food. It is a complete change of eating pattern and it sounds difficult to follow in starting. But gradually it becomes easy, it is one of the magical diet-plan that helps to lose weight and improve health without counting the calories. However, according to the health advisors, before starting the intermittent fasting it is essential to consult the doctor, so take the proper advice and follow the respective instructions to get the quick and appropriate outcomes.

Chapter 8
Intermittent Fasting And Workout

"It's important to note that our fasting window should be tailored around our workout regimen."
Demmy James

Fasting is the diet and meal strictness that a person follows throughout a day without cutting and counting on the calories. People do the fasting for the weight loss, to maintain the overall health and to get the fitness benefits, etc. Intermittent fasting is the new and completely modified form of diet that gets popularity among people, due to multiple of reasons. Some people believe to still follow the workout with the intermittent fasting schedule.

It's not something which can hurt your health, it's just a change in plan to have a meal during the days. There are multiple ways that people adopt to follow the diet, as well as during intermittent fasting it is completely safe to have workouts. The intensity of your workout should be adjustable and as per the health expert advice. According to the research and fitness expert, if you follow the intermittent fasting, then try not to follow the workout with that in parallel. When you are on fasting, the body is already in a position of active metabolism process and workout also boosts the metabolic function. So, combining the both things together may lead to a crash and may not be good for everyone.

On the other hand, people who are following the intermittent fasting and parallel start working out may see significant effects in weight loss. Consequently, it improves the fitness as well as stamina or leads a high level of losing the fats and reduces weight. Workout utilizes energy and muscles take it from the stored body fats and after that the body requires calories to rebuild. So, it is necessary for the intermittent fasting followers that consume more water during or after workout, in order to keep the body hydrated. You can use some kind of electrolyte while doing the exercise as well.

Both fasting and working out together not only improve the metabolism, but is also good for the overall digestive process. The body absorbs more energy and improves the blood circulation that revitalizes the cells and actives the parts of body where the blood or nutrients are not fully supplied, due to inactivity. With intermittent fasting you can have a whole food snacks, instead of having pre-workout meals, because they are good in energy supply and deliver healthy amount of proteins and carbs into the body.

Fasting And Gain Muscle

Usually, people think and consider that the fasting is the way to lose weight, as well as muscle mass. Thinking in different paradigm, like maintain or gain muscle with intermittent fasting is relatively difficult so, in this process, people put themselves into a strict diet plan and follow limited meal program to get the appropriate results. Limited calorie intake and meal window help to lose weight and to get the lean muscle mass, but is not possible for the muscle gain. For the muscle gain a person needs to consume more calories with the workout that stimulates the tissues growth and increases in overall muscle mass.

Weight training in fasting

Weight trainings are good for the muscle strength and for improving overall stamina. It puts a person metabolism in an active position that leads healthier lifestyle. Intermittent fasting significantly affects the overall weight reduction quickly so, doing the weight training with the fasting, may help to prevent the loss of muscle mass. As per the training professional and health expert, it is highly recommended to do the weight training with the fasting way to lose weight and strengthen the muscles.

Safety tips during exercise with fasting

Generally, research supports well to fasting and working out together, but to have great and effective outcomes, it is necessary to follow the way in an appropriate manner that just decreases the weight, not the health, such as doing the exercise with fasting but following the safety tips to combine them in a safe way. Here are some safety tips a person should follow during workouts with intermittent fasting:

In fasting meal timing plays an important role, fitness expert suggests to take a meal close to your workout intensity; this, not only help to fuel up the body with energy, but you can also enjoy the better results with your high intensity workouts.

It is known that during the training it is important to keep the body hydrated, so consume more water during the fasting time and use some electrolytes, which are low calorie source to fuel up muscles and tissues, instead of any energy drink or a workout drink.

Working out with intermittent fasting is good, but parallel a person needs to listen up the body first, as if you follow a high intensity exercise and you feel a kind of exertion, then take a break because it is important.

Build or maintain muscles

Intermittent fasting gives the fastest result way of dieting, as long as it is an exceptional way, not like a random method to lose weight. People follow a meal window as per their requirement and fast for a certain time or day in a week; it not only helps to improve the health but is good for losing weight effectively. If you add fasting with working out, the results will be multiplying by two. Remember that the fasting and exercise together just help to give muscle strength and they give quick results, but for gaining the mass it is not an appropriate way because, to gain muscle, usually a person needs to consume more calorie and then burns it through workout. By combining the intermittent fasting with the workout only give a way to maintain the muscle mass and strengthen them.

Effects On Men & Women Physique

Intermittent fasting is considered as the best way to lose weight and control over the obesity. It is one of the most popular diet-plan that is getting popular, due to its unique and remarkable benefits. If we talk about the effects of the intermittent fasting on men & women, then, according to the studies, it is reported that both have different results and experiences while following the fasting. This is because the hormones and the behaviors change, as well as the results and responses of the body towards the same phenomena.

Women struggles more than men

According to the study, it is reviewed that women struggle more than men in losing the weight and to get the lean muscle mass, because the hormonal changes and chemical reactions are totally changed in both of them. So, intermittent fasting, strict diet and workout plans affect the hormones production and can influence the fertility and reproduction more in women than in men. The women internal system is more sensitive than men's and effects the muscle mass while losing the weight. It can increase the chances of improper ovulation cycle that can disturbed the hormonal balance and cycle.

Why women face hormonal deficiencies?

While following the intermittent fasting, women face the hormonal deficiency that may cause multiple of health complications like indigestion problem, disturbed menstruation cycle and effect, due to the loss of muscle mass with the weight and fats. Other than a man, a woman faces more problems because she's not able to take the proteins and, due to strict diet and meal plans, hormonal changes occur and affect them more rapidly.

There are multiple of reasons a woman can face problems with fasting, like:

- Low level of nutrients and consumption of the food may cause the nutrients deficiency.
- If a woman follows tight and high intensity workouts with the fasting, they are followed the too much stress and exertion.

- It can be due to limited time for the recovery and rest between the workouts and fasting breakouts.
- Low level of the intake can affect the immune system and raise the chances of illness like flu, fever, infection and others.

How stress influence health and hormonal level?

When a person on the low carbs and calorie diet, has to definitely face multiple of hormonal and behavioral changes. Sometimes people are too aggressive towards the following of the intermittent fasting meal window with the exercise, so the result is stress and undue pressure to lose weight quickly that significantly affect their ability to fight against the upcoming challenges. High level of stress hormones production disturbs the balance of hormonal level and disturbs overall function abruptly.

The most important thing in this situation that has to be considered is consulting the health consultant and making a meal plan accordingly. Be consistent in following the plan, do not stress out to get quick results, listen to your body and act accordingly. Eat the healthy and nutritional food with the low or high intensity workout and follow the guideline of the instructor and health consultant to avoid the issue.

Best Exercise During Intermittent Fasting

Workout is the best way to keep yourself active, as well as it has a vital effect on the person's overall health. With regular exercise you can not only enjoy a fresh and lively lifestyle, but also it boosts the metabolism function. By an improved blood circulation many health complications can be deal in a better way. If a person follows a diet plan to lose weight, then combining the workout could significantly impact the overall results; even the researchers recommend that intermittent fasting can be more useful and beneficial if it is followed by a proper schedule exercise. It can be high or low intensity trainings as per the person's capability and requirements.

The choice of the trainings depends on the method of intermittent fasting that a person chooses to lose weight. In general, it's just a followed meal plans a person adopts for a day to lose the excessive weight, so it does not only improve the health but it also elicits other complications that can influence a person's life, due to obesity.

Workout timings with fasting

For the right and fruitful results, it is necessary to follow the right way to involve the workout plans. For example, some people follow the two times working out routine with the intermittent fasting and others have one; this depends on the method you choose for fasting and the intensity you want to have to get the results, so the morning time is considered an appropriate time to work out with fasting.

Build your own workout routine

You can follow or build your own workout routine as well; aforementioned, it depends on what you are expecting from your body to be followed. Some people want to lean muscle mass and reduce the size, others are looking to reduce the fats or weight by gaining the muscle mass. You can build or design your own workout routine that entirely depends on the priority you are looking for. Firstly, for the muscle mass adopt the weight training with the cardio sessions and consume more proteins that give strength to the muscle. Secondly, for strength deadlifts, push-ups, dips, pull ups and squats are considered effective workouts for women and men as well.

Weight trainings with fasting

Weight training with intermittent fasting is an effective option because it will not only help to lose weight, but it will also improve the stamina, strength for the muscle growth. Sometimes people may lose the muscle weight while following the intermittent fasting plans, so the weight training will keep the muscle in shape and do not let you lose the mass.

Cardio session with fasting

Cardio sessions are not only effective for weight lose but also help to improve the blood circulation throughout the body. These sessions help to keep a person active and considered more effective to have a good stamina and strength; with fasting it will help to improve the overall metabolic process and reduce inflammation in blood and body.

Cardiovascular exercises

Cardiovascular trainings are effective and can be done anywhere like at gym or at home; you do not need a special gym equipment. These trainings are effective and 25 times more effective then pulling and pushing weights. Leg raises, crunches, squats, push-ups, pull-ups etc. are effective and influential trainings that can be done with fasting to get the healthier outcomes.

Chapter 9
Tips For Successful Transformation

"Fitness is the relationship that you cannot think it works after cheating" & *"your body can do it but the time is just to convince your mind"* - *Unknown*

Losing weight and being back in the ideal physique is a challenging job for people who are dealing with the obesity issue. But in reality, there is nothing that cannot be possible in real life. As a matter of fact, there are multiple of diet plans and health tips that are really helpful and impressive to give the outcomes with no side effects. Intermittent fasting is considered one of them, it is not like any other traditional way to diet and lose fats, as it provides a meal window between the fasting: eating and fasting are divided in between the whole day. This method boosts metabolism and helps to transform the body.

If you are one of those who is tired of the weight and fats or wants to lose them effectively to be back in a good shape, then intermittent fasting is the appropriate and impressive way to be active and fit without any health side effects. It is getting popular because it provides ease and comfort in life with the simple window of fasting and eating in a day. According to the health professionals, it is important to follow the procedure for at least one or two months continuously, without any break.

People who followed the fasting methods talked about this proudly and discussed their body transformation. To achieve the ideal and fit body with lean muscle mass, it is necessary to follow some impressive tips and procedure that will not only help to reduce the weight, as well strengthen the overall muscle mass with the strong and impressive way.

Motivational Success Stories

Losing weight and being back in the fit and slim physique is quite difficult and tough. There are multiple of people around us who tried multiple ways to do that but failed. Losing weight is not something a magic can happen to anyone in a day or weeks, it leads a continues change or lifestyle change that brings hope and transformation. Intermittent fasting is getting popular among people around the world just because of its remarkable benefits and long-term benefits in a person's life.

If we just look around, we can easily find multiple success stories, who just tried and lost weight with following the intermittent fasting meal windows. Here we have some for you to just give a motivation and inspiration to follow:

1. James Kevin

By profession James is a doctor, he guides others about the health, fitness and leading good lifestyle, but due to his unwanted eating habits and food choice made him fat. He even did not think to get back into to shape, then an incident happened in his life that changed everything completely. His sister died with a serious chronical disease, right at that movement he realized that he had an option. Indeed, with the intermittent fasting he put himself in the stick schedule of eating vegetables and low carbs food product and followed a proper workout session parallel to the fasting; the results were amazing in just 18 months: he lost around 125 pounds.

"I am amazed with the results, there are diets that give results but intermittent fasting is medically an amazing one. That's why I choose this and see the difference." James Kevin

2. Jane Wright

Being a mother is no doubt a blessing, but a person has to go along with the whole process of fighting for the weight loss. Jane got a lot of weight after having a baby and tried multiple ways to reduce but failed. The motivation she had to be the perfect and fit mother by physique, as well as her daughter can be proud of her. With the weight of 337 pounds she just started the intermitted fasting 21-day meal plan. Parallel to this, she added the 30 minutes cardio training session into her routine that went for the high intensity workouts. She fasted for almost 16 hours a day and only eat 8 hours; with all her effects and dedication, she just lost the 105 pounds in 12 months. She shared her excitement: "I am happy and motivated and found quality time with my daughter like never before. With this, all I have patience and consistency, which are the keys to achieve any of your goals."

3. Hunter Hobbs

He is a man with weight of almost 200 pounds with the height of 5 feet 10 inches. He found himself overweight and decided to choose the meal plan of intermittent fasting, with the continuous effort of three months, the consistent fasting, eating meal windows and workouts he almost lost the 42 pounds. He takes picture of himself every day and tracks his all way of transformation together. He just lost the almost 42 pounds in three months with the intermittent fasting meal plans.

He was excited and he shared his review, "I am surprised and amazed with the results of this intermittent fasting. I just started following this by getting the inspiration from the multiple people who shared their success stories. This gave me encouragement to make myself as an inspiration for someone."

4. Brittany May

Brittany May was a woman with the weight of 514 pounds and she was getting hard for her to handle it all together. She heard about the intermittent fasting meal plans and she chose the one for herself. With the continuous effort of following the diet plan and exercise, she reduced almost 336 pounds in the period of two years. It is an incredible achievement as May said, "I actually want to lose the stubborn body weight and change my lifestyle to enjoy the pleasure of lifestyle and relationship, now finally I got what I want to get." Losing weight not only transformed her life, but also gave her a new direction to drive it on her own way.

5. Ria Reed

Intermittent fasting proven the best and most comfortable way to lose weight and get lean muscle mass. Ria lost almost 32 pounds with the transformed body mass; thanks to the intermitted fasting, with the high intensity cardio session and weight trainings, she did not only achieve her target, but she also felt confident about sharing her transformation path.

She shares that the "the family holidays become memorable and more than expectations than I never had in dreams before."

6. Kelly and Mike

Losing weight together is a couple goals that is proved by Kelly and Mike. Both give motivation to each other's and started the intermittent fasting together. At the starting time Kelly was with the weight of 219 pounds and Mike have weight 259 pounds. After eating or fasting with 21 days' meal plan and exercise, both lost some remarkable pounds like Kelly lost 57 pounds and Mike lost 58 pounds. That was an incredible change for both of them, so that they shared their motivational and transformation story together.

Tips For Transformation

While following the fasting, people achieve their body transformation target with the impressive way within time. According to the experiences of different people, multiple things are really important and they boost the process to achieve the targets really quickly.

Transformation needs the working and strict to the plan with the proper discipline and dedication. If you follow fasting, it does not mean you do not need planning. Making strategy and the implementation of a right plan to achieve right outcomes is an important and necessary option.

Here we have some impressive tips for those who are new and want to follow the transformation procedure to get an impressive body.

Remove junk food

Most important thing that a person has to consider for the body transformation, is that she / he has to remove all the junk food from the house, because fasting, initially, makes it is difficult to fight from the hunger, and in case of hunger attack there are probabilities to consume the junk, if they are in approach. So, replace the junk food with the healthy snacks and whole food that are full of protein and low in carbs, this it helps to make your stomach feel full for a longer time and makes things easier at the time of the fasting.

Interact socially

If you are facing problem with fighting obesity in its best way, then it is important to fight and interact with the social circle, for example: ask friends, family and other close ones to how and what to follow for the transformation, because around us it is easy to find out the impressive stories of people who have done lots of efforts on themselves, and their experiences could support other people.

Start reading about food and health

Reading will definitely give impressive ideas and awareness about the things in totally different way. Firstly, for the successful transformation a person needs to start reading about the other's successful stories to get the motivation. Secondly, a person needs to find out more about the food and things that helps to boost metabolism and what to avoid if someone wants to achieve a desired fit and slim physique.

Have picture before starting

The necessary thing before starting the fasting or any other method of diet is to take a picture and save it as a record; this will give a motivation to go long on the way of fasting or dieting, and helps to track the performance too.

Be consistent with plan

Consistency is more than necessary in the way that a person chooses to go along with, as it is not about that you just start for some time and then switch to another plan. So, for the intermittent fasting, it is important to at least try the method for one or two months consecutively.

Bring changes into workout routine

Workout really helps in the whole transformation process, it gives muscles strength and put the body in the process of continuous fat reduction. If a person is following a low and simple intensity workout, then it is necessary to move towards the high intensity workout schedule and modify the trainings. Consequently, you can add the weight trainings and high intensity cardio trainings in the whole routine to get the better outcomes.

Plan and prepare meal

Consume more green vegetables and protein in your daily intake with the exercise and other activities; try to prepare the whole food with low fats and low carbs options. Watching out on the fat intake is another important thing for the transformation, use the nuts as a source of good fats, but check the calories you are consuming in your eating time.

Improve the self-control

During the whole process of fasting or dieting the difficult things is to keep the check on the hand and the choice of having the meals all around, as long as a person may face the episodes of the hunger and craving. Thus, improve your self-control over the junk by choosing the healthy and low carbs food option and switch to whole food instead of high carbs, and so on. Furthermore, clean your snacks choices or meal at the time of eating so you can survive best at the time of fasting.

Keep yourself hydrated

Hydration is the most important consideration; during workouts and meal plans consume more water and low calories drinks options. Water helps to keep up the metabolism that actively boosts the process of fat reduction and helps in transformation. So, tea, coffee, electrolytes and other non-sugary drinks can be consumed in the fasting or with the eating schedule as well.

Manage stress

Stress can be a hurdle in the whole process of transformation. Thus, it is important to reduce the stress and keep the control on it, because it could affect the process of weight loss and fats reduction. Lastly, to lower the stress, try to have good amount of sleep and rest after workouts and between the exercises.

Set goals and share

Without goals, setting the process cannot be measured so fast. To get the impressive transformation try to make a defined goal, such as short term goals and share them with your social circle; this will help to keep up the motivational level and a courage to achieve them in the short time period.

Whatever the procedure you are following for the transformation like intermittent fasting or any other diet plan, the important thing is to keep following with a consistent time period. Consistency is the key to achieve any of the goal, whether it is related to the health and fitness target. Intermittent fasting is getting popular because of its impressive and outstanding results that are not only to reduce the weight, but also to give multiple other health benefits.

Chapter 10
Women And Intermittent Fasting

Intermittent fasting is the most popular method if you want to get the lean muscle mass and to reduce the weight. A person who is following this way to diet have a more energetic and motivated journey to lose weight. Intermittent fasting will defiantly give multiple health benefits, no matter you are a man or a woman. The important consideration is just that every person has different biological structure, so things will work differently for everyone. Some can get the results quickly and others have to stay and consistent for a little longer to get the results. But generally, it is the safe and best way to lose weight. However, according to the multiple research, the intermittent fasting is highly recommendable for men but not for women.

Intermittent fasting is a bit technical method that works by engaging the body in the process of absorbing and digestion of food into the body and keeps the body fuel up for the whole time of fasting. Besides, it accelerates the process of fats burning in the state of fasting; in simple words, fasting is the period that usually there are around 12, 16 or 18 hours of fasting, in which you should not have food or just consume water or low- calorie drinks like green tea, coffee or tea without sugar and milk. Usually people have the meal window of around 8 hours or 6 hours a day and the rest of the time spend on fasting.

What's good with intermittent fasting?

Intermittent fasting is an effective result and is oriented to diet and to lose weight, by giving remarkable good outcomes, which are:

- Loss weight and it helps to maintain the healthy one
- With this it is easy to get the lean muscle mass and muscle strength as well
- A person can feel energetic and can control over the junk food
- It can increase the insulin sensitivity and reduce the inflammation
- It also helps to enhance the overall cognitive function

Intermittent fasting sounds tricky for women

In general, intermittent fasting is an impressive and technical thing to lose weight but for women it is a way different thing. It happens because the woman system is different from man's and production or responses of the hormones to a certain scenario is totally changed. The intense fasting with the workout not only leans the muscle mass, but it also makes changes in hormones. Especially, it affects directly on the fertility hormones and ovulation process. Due to hormonal disturbance a woman can experience multiple health issues like:

- Irregular menstruation cycle

- Metabolic stress and anxiety
- Fertility issues
- Ovulation disturbance
- Difficult to take enough or good sleep
- Ovaries can be shrinking and make difficult to conceive

If a woman wants to follow the intermittent fasting then most importantly, make sure to follow the relax and different fasting and eating approach. It can be convenient if the method must be chosen after consulting the health consultant, so the hormones function will not be disturbed.

During Mensuration

For a woman it is technical and crucial to follow a diet plan to lose the weight, as compared to men. Because both have different hormones and behaviors of the hormones that respond differently in different situations. In general studies it is not sure that the intermittent fasting can cause problems with the menstruation cycle, but it can in some cases. In fasting usually people lower the calories intake that turns it an effective way to overcome the metabolic problem and reduce the weight; nonetheless, causing issue with the periods does not just happen because of the intermittent fasting.

According to some studies, it is discussed that the intermittent fasting can influence the periods in a woman, if the calorie intake reduces up to a drastic low level, because fasting puts the body in the high metabolic process and, due to lower calorie diet and narrow eating window, it effects the hormones production. Finally, imbalance hormones directly influence the fertility and menstruation.

The important thing that need to be considered while following intermittent fasting is add nutrients in your eating window like nuts, fruits, green leafy vegetables and a lot of healthy snacks, as long as they will keep the body function streamline to act properly, and they also help to control over the exertion and stressful condition that can influence the hormonal balance badly.

For Pregnancy & Breastfeeding

In women, hormones are interconnected and influence by the intense internal deficiencies that can cause low calorie intake or low nutritional food supply to the cells and body parts; with intermittent fasting, metabolism function goes high and utilizes the internal stored energy to keep the energy level up. However, if due to intense fasting and exertion hormones got disturbed, they lead to the disturbance in the digestion, metabolism, blood pressure or blood sugar level as well. So, the adverse situation can be the cause of infertility, improper periods session or other fertility issues.

Health consultant does not suggest the intermittent fasting to those women who is trying to conceive or pregnant ones. As well as breastfeeding mothers, they should follow the intermittent fasting because it can affect the nutrients and energy components that are essential for a child in the early ages.

Losing weight is good, but a person needs to listen up the body first, such as for pregnant and breastfeeding women, it is not suitable to mess up with the hormonal production just to lose the weight.

During Menopause

Menopause is the process that a woman has to face and goes through in the early age like around 40 or 50. During the process multiple health and hormonal changes take place inside the body that effect the body structure and hormonal changes equally.

What Is menopause?

It is a period that a woman does not have periods for the entire year or more than that, it happens when the ovaries stop producing the eggs. Usually, an average ratio of menopause occurs at the age of 45 or 51 years; it is considered as a hard time and multiple health complications can affect a woman, for instance: a woman is not able to conceive when the procedure begins and gradually stops the periods that leads high level of hormonal and behavioral changes.

How menopause effect a woman life?

During the process of menopause, the body produces limited amount of progesterone or testosterone hormones. High level of hormonal changes can have multiple effects on a person's life, such as:

- Gaining weight and fats quickly
- Facing the stress and high level of anxiety
- Due to low testosterone sex driving can be affected, as well as facing vaginal dryness
- Sometime facing hair loss, mood swings and dry skin issues

- Insomnia and restless sleeping

Menopause and weight

Menopause directly affects the weight, usually it is noticed that woman gains weight quickly, due to the certain body and hormonal changes in the body. Furthermore, there are multiple other factors that can influence the overall health, such as the increase in weight that can develop the risk of obesity and high blood pressure. Parallel, it may have disturbed the blood glucose level in the body that can increase the risk of diabetes.

Due to certain complications and problems, doctors highly recommend to control over the weight gain and try to adopt the ways to reduce it with the optimal level, by means of proper schedule diet and workout sessions that can only give opportunity to control the weight and other associated issues. A hormonal test is recommended as well.

Intermitted fasting in menopause

Intermittent fasting is the tested and highly recommended way to lose the weight and it restores the energy and stamina. It is followed by extended the time between the meals and fasting, as the glucose is the primary source of the energy that your body needs to function properly. While with fasting, the body is not able to get the glucose from the food and it starts getting it from the stored body fats; in the end, it gradually starts burning the fats and utilizes that energy to spend the hours of fasting.

Health consultants consider that a woman during the menopause can adopt the intermittent fasting technique to lose weight and to fuel up the body energy, for the reason that it does not only keep you out of stress, but it also manages the insulin level, reduces inflammation and is good for the overall cognitive function. The ideal hours of fasting for a day is 16 hours or 12 hours and between the meal window of 6 hours or 8 hours; During the eating time it is important to consume excessive water, as well as during the fasting time.

The Best Methods Of Intermittent Fasting For Women

Intermittent fasting is considered a technical concept that needs a lot of effort to measure the exact fasting and eating ratio, so the health complications can be avoided. Experts said that the intensity of fasting for women cannot be the same as for men, this is because each of them has different hormonal functions that leads in a body differently. As well as the biological structure of both of them is totally different from each other, so, it is important to avoid the fasting, if you may face the serious health complication and, due to any reason, face some significant side effects.

Tips to adopt for fasting

By considering the health and hormonal changes a woman has to follow the tips that are designed and prescribed by the experts. It includes:

- Try not to follow the intense fasting schedule like do not fast for more than 24 hours at once.
- The best time zone and schedule to fast is 12 hours or probably 16 hours

- Do not fast for consecutive days in the first two or three weeks of fasting, always try to indulge with the alternative days for fasting.
- Keep your self-hydrated during the whole fasting time and follow the good nutritional food to break-fast.
- Do not go for the intense training or the weight trainings, especially in the days of fasting, the best training sessions are like yoga, light cardio, walking or running which are the appropriate options.
- Break your fast if you feel dizziness or any unpleasant feeling during the fasting.
- Keep yourself fuel up in eating hours with the good fats like nuts, low carb diet and proteins, because they are good in weight loss, as well as maintain the hormonal balance.

There are multiple of fasting methods that are common and popular among the people, but due to the biological structure differences, every method is not appropriate for women. However, that doesn't mean a woman cannot fast to lose weight, though there are some effective and useful ways that are feasible and appropriate for them. Plus, they do not harm the hormonal balances and they never cause the fertility issues.

Here are some methods for the safe intermittent fasting for women:

16:8 method

This is one of the most popular and common method of intermittent fasting. The method is also known as the lean-gains method. This way not only helps to reduce the weight but it is also effective to get the lean muscle mass.

This method is considered completely safe for the women. Finally, in this intermittent fasting, an individual follows the 16 hours of having fast and 6 hours for eating throughout a day.

24-hour protocol

It is another effective and safe intermitted fasting method for women that usually follows just twice in a week: it is also known as eat-stop-eat fasting type. Usually in this fasting type a person does not have any eating window and has to follow the 24 hours of fast. According to the health consultant for woman, it is necessary to just follow this method twice a week, but more than that may be not good for the health.

5:2 diet plan

5:2 diet plan is the fast diet in which a person has to divide the meal into two equal parts with just 500 calorie consumption in a day. This diet is just followed two days in a week and rest of the day you can take normal food. This fast diet is considered the safe one for both men and women. You can have two days with the meal of 500 calories for each day and the rest of five days a week follow the normal diet.

Chapter 11: Recipes

Raspberry Power Pancake

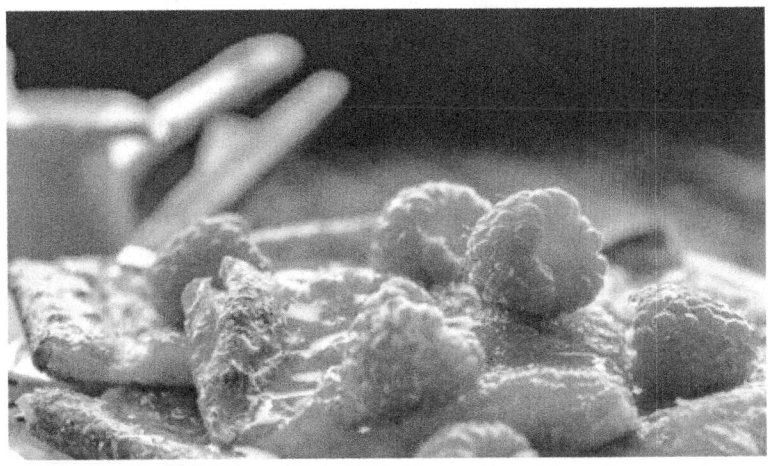

Preparation time: 05 minutes I **Cooking time**: 15 minutes I **Servings**: 4

Ingredients:
- 1 egg
- 1 and 1/3 cups flour
- ¼ teaspoon vanilla extract
- 2 tablespoons
- melted butter
- 1 ½ cups milk
- ½ teaspoon salt

- 3 teaspoons baking powder

- 2 tablespoons vegetable oil
- 1 tablespoon ground sugar

- 1 cup raspberries

Directions: Mix egg, milk, vanilla extract, and butter in a bowl. Mix flour, salt and baking powder in another bowl. Now add these mixed dry ingredients into the egg batter. Mix it well and leave it for 5 minutes. Preheat the pan on medium flame. Grease the pan with vegetable oil. Pour the 1/4th batter into the pan and add raspberries at the top. Cook it for few minutes until bubbles start to appear. Now flip it and cook the other side for 2 minutes. Sprinkle the grounded sugar on the pancakes.

Nutrition: Protein 8g, Calories 329, Fat 14g, Carbohydrate 46g.

Chocolate Chip Whey Waffles

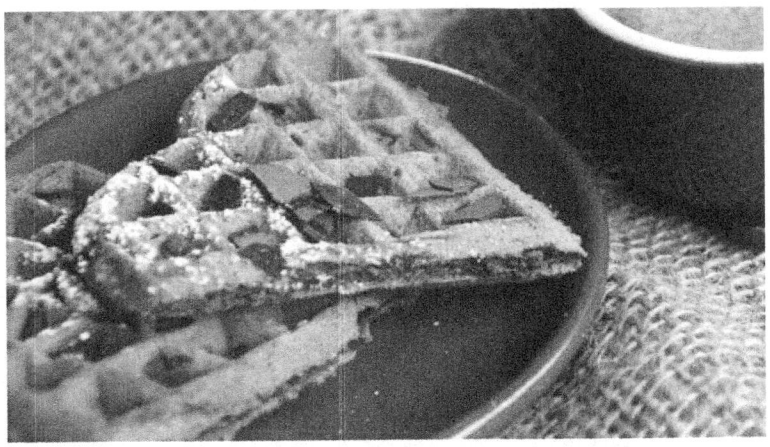

Preparation time: 10 minutes / **Cooking time**: 10 minutes / **Servings**: 2

Ingredients:
- 2 eggs
- 1 tablespoon baking powder
- 2 tablespoons coconut flour
- 2 scoop chocolate whey protein
- ½ tablespoon vanilla extract
- 1 tablespoon coconut sugar
- 1 tablespoon chocolate chips

Directions:
Preheat the greased waffle iron. In a bowl mix flour, protein powder, sugar, and baking powder. Now add rest of the ingredients in the dry mixture and mix them until all the ingredients combined properly. Now put the batter in the preheated waffle iron and cook for approximately 4 minutes.

Serve it immediately by adding some chocolate chips on its top.

Nutrition: Protein 28g, fat 9g, Carbohydrate 25g, Calories 292, Sugar 14g, Cholesterol 228mg.

Cinnamon Sugar Donuts

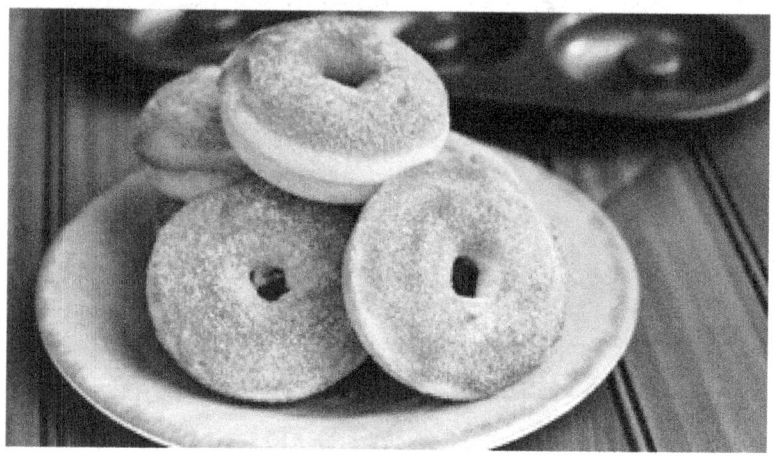

Preparation time: 10 minutes *| Cooking time*: 10 minutes *| Servings*: 2

Ingredients:
- ½ cup sugar
- 1 ½ cups flour
- ½ teaspoon salt
- ½ cup milk
- ½ teaspoons cinnamon
- ½ teaspoon nutmeg
- 1 egg
- 1 tablespoon melted butter
- 2 teaspoons baking powder

Directions:
Put the mix the salt, flour, nutmeg, baking powder, and cinnamon in a bowl. Take another bowl and mix all the remaining ingredients. Now combine the wet ingredients in the dry ingredients and whisk them well. Take a pan with oil and put the batter in the form of donuts in the oil. Fry these donuts on the medium flame. And serve it immediately.

Nutrition: Protein 3.6g, Fat 8.1g, Carbohydrate 34.3g, Calories 222, Sugar 18.6g, Cholesterol 47mg.

Poached Eggs & Avocado

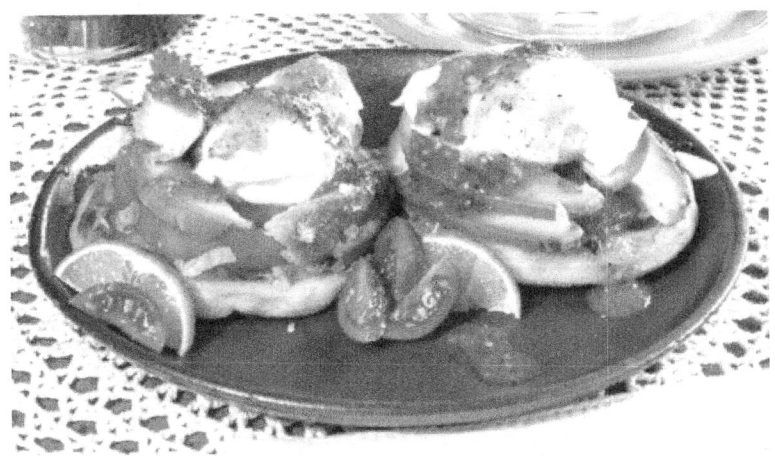

Preparation time: 10 minutes I Cooking time: 10 minutes I Servings: 2

Ingredients:
- 2 slices of bread
- 2 eggs
- A pinch of salt and black pepper

- 2 tablespoons sheared cheese
- 1/3 smashed avocado
- ½ cup fresh herbs
- ½ cup cubed cut tomatoes

Directions:

Take a pot to boil the water. Boil the water and turn off the heat. Now carefully crack the eggs in the boiled water. Cover the pot for around 4 to 5 minutes. Toast the bread slices and set the avocado on it. Take out the eggs carefully with the help of a spatula and place it on the toast. Sprinkle salt, pepper, cheese, tomato, and fresh herbs on the egg. And it is ready to serve.

Nutrition: Protein 23.3g, Fats 20.4g, Calories 393, Sugar 5.7g, Cholesterol 34.6mg.

Chocolate Chia Plain Pudding

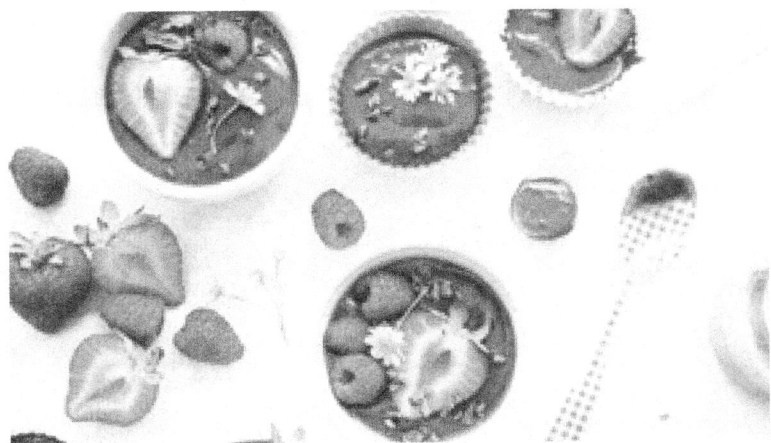

Preparation time: 05 minutes I **Chilling time**: 4 hours I **Servings**: 2

Ingredients:
- 1/3 cup chia seeds
- 1 cup coconut or almond milk
- ¼ cup cocoa powder

- ½ teaspoon vanilla extract
- 2 tablespoons maple syrup

- ½ cup Seasonal Berries (optional)

Directions:
Take a bowl and add all the ingredients in it. Mix all the ingredients until they merged in a proper way. Check the sweet and if required add more syrup in it to make it according to your taste. Now place it in the refrigerator for at least 4 hours for chilling. Serve it by adding berries on its top.

Nutrition: Protein 6g, Fats 20.4g, Calories 164, Sugar 1g, Carbohydrates 14g.

Gluten-Free Pumpkin Pancake

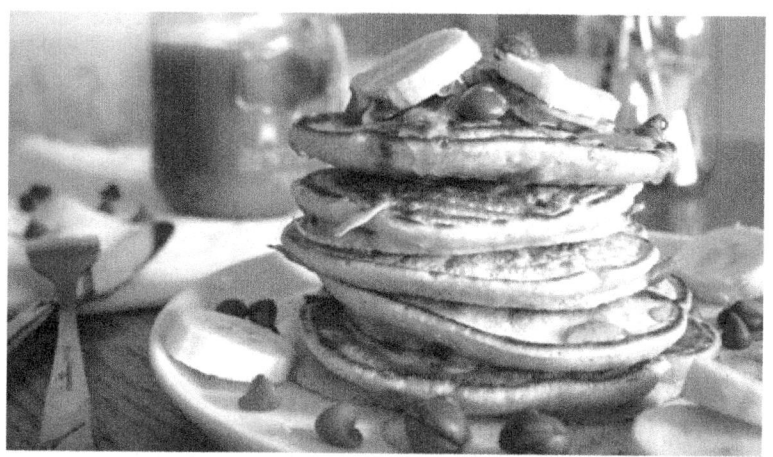

*Preparation time: 15 minutes I **Cooking time:** 10 minutes I **Servings:** 15*

Ingredients:
- 2 eggs
- 1½ cups low-fat milk
- 2 tablespoons melted butter

- ½ cup pumpkin pure
- 2 teaspoons pumpkin pie spice
- 1 teaspoon vanilla extract
- 1½ cups gluten free pancake mix

Directions:

Mix eggs, milk, pumpkin puree, and butter in a bowl. Add pancake mix in it gradually and mix it well, salt and baking powder in another bowl. Now add the remaining ingredients and mix well. Put a greased skillet over medium heat and pour better in it. Cook it until its color turned into gold. Cook on both sides and serve it immediately.

Nutrition: Protein 3g, Calories 113, Fat 3g, Carbohydrate 19g, Sugar 5g.

Roasted Sweet Potato & Poblano Tacos

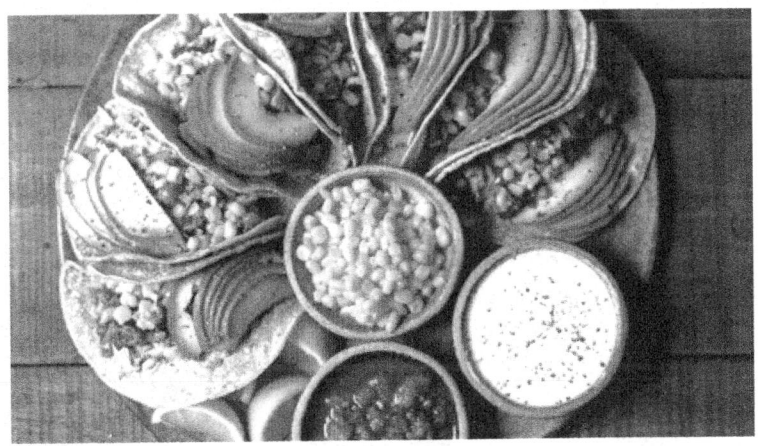

Preparation time: 15 minutes | Cooking time: 45 minutes | Servings: 2

Ingredients:
- 3 eggs
- 1 cubes sweet potato
- 1 thin sliced pepper bells
- 1 cup corns
- 4 tortillas
- ½ diced avocado

- ½ teaspoon crushed salt and black pepper
- roasted Tomatillo salsa

Directions:
Preheat the oven at 450F and prepare the baking dish with paper. Roast the salsa and vegetables for 15 minutes into the preheated oven. Now reduce the oven temperature to 425F. Take 2 baking dishes add potatoes in one. And other vegetables in the second. Drizzle oil, salt, and pepper on it and baked potatoes for 25 minutes and vegetables for 15 minutes. Cook eggs and scrambled them. In the serving dish add everything and serve with salsa.

Nutrition: Protein 8g, Fat 12g, Carbohydrate 55g, Calories 350, Sugar 10g

Sugar-Free Oatmeal Cookies

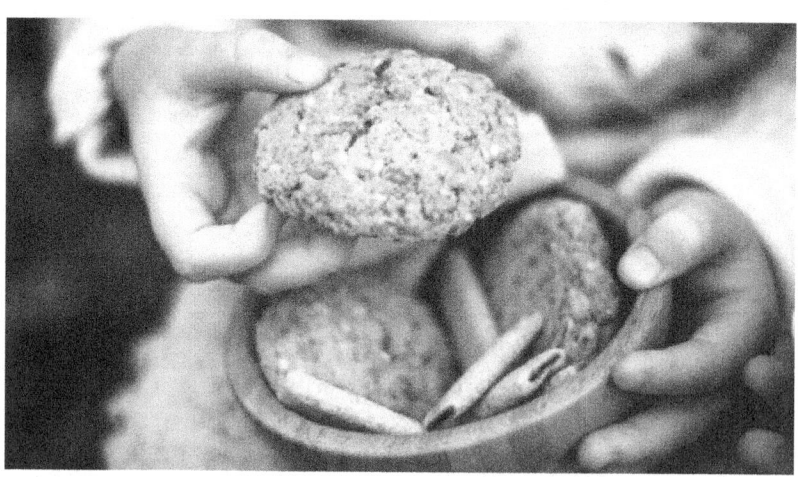

*Preparation time: 10 minutes I **Cooking time**: 10 minutes I **Servings**: 15*

Ingredients:

- ½ cup butter
- 2 eggs
- 1 ¼ rolled oats
- 1 teaspoon almond flour
- 1 teaspoon cinnamon
- 1 sugar-free baking powder
- ¼ teaspoon salt
- 1 teaspoon vanilla extract
- ¾ cup of gluten sugar

Directions:

Preheat the oven at 350F and prepare a baking tray with a liner. Take a bowl and combine the eggs, butter and gluten sugar and mix well. Now mix the remaining ingredients in it and mix well. Add some water if required to thin the batter so that all the ingredients merged well. Now scoop the batter in the tray and baked it for 10 minutes. It is ready to serve.

Nutrition: Protein 3g, Fat 8g, Calories 103g, Carbohydrates 5g, Sugar 0.4g

Egg Muffin With Broccoli

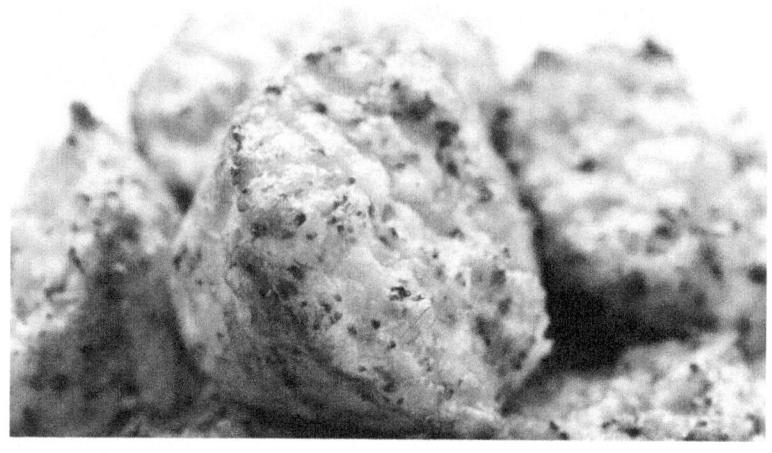

Preparation time: 05 minutes / **Cooking time**: 15 minutes / **Servings**: 12

Ingredients:
- 1 teaspoon salt
- 10 eggs
- ½ teaspoon black pepper
- ½ teaspoon garlic powder
- ½ teaspoon thyme
- 2/3 cup grated cheese
- 1½ cups steamed and chopped broccoli

Directions:
Prepare 12 muffin cups with liner and preheat the oven at 400F temperature. Take a bowl and beat the eggs thoroughly. Now add the remaining ingredients in it by adding cheese and broccoli in the last. Mix all the ingredients until they merged well. Pour the batter in the prepared muffin cups

evenly. Bake it for 12 to 15 minutes and serve it immediately.

Nutrition: Protein 6g, Fats 5g, Calories 82, Cholesterol 142mg.

Banana Blueberry Muffins

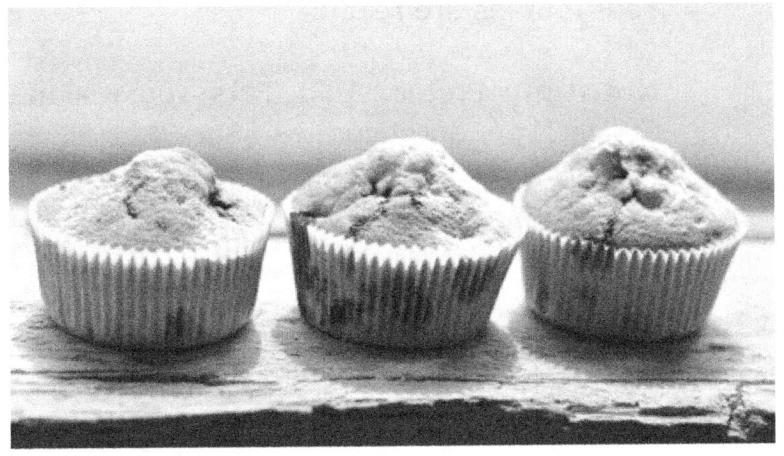

Preparation time: *10 minutes* | **Cooking time**: *20 minutes* | **Servings**: *12*

Ingredients:
- 1 egg
- 1/2 cup mashed banana
- ¼ cup vegetable oil

- 2/3 cup milk
- 2/3 cup gluten sugar

- 2½ cup teaspoons baking powder
- 2 cups flour

- 1 cup well drained blueberries

Directions: Take a bowl and add all the ingredients except blueberries. Stir it well until all the ingredients merged. In the end, add blueberries in it and fold it in the mixture. Prepare the 12 muffin cups with liner. Pour the batter equally in the cups. Put the cups in the 400F temperature preheated oven for 18 to 20 minutes. Your muffins are ready.

Nutrition: Protein 4.5g, Fats 10g, Calories 332, Sugar 31g, Carbohydrates 58g.

Energetic Lunch Recipes

Grilled Cheeseburger

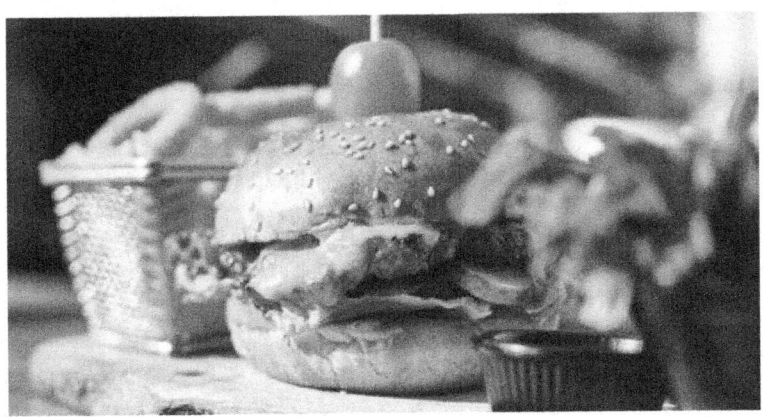

*Preparation time: 15 minutes | **Cooking time**: 15 minutes | **Servings**: 4*

Ingredients:

- 2 chopped tomatoes
- 1 tablespoon olive oil
- 1 cup taco seasoning
- 3 tablespoons unsalted butter
- 1 ½ cup grated cheese
- 8 slices wheat bread
- ½ teaspoon salt and black pepper
- 1 pound ground beef

Directions: Put a skillet with oil over the medium flame. Cook the beef by adding salt and pepper in it for 5 minutes until it cooked well. Add cheese, tomato, and seasoning in it and cook it for about 1 minute until cheese melted. Take the bread and apply butter on it and grill it. Now spread the beef better on the 4 slices evenly and add cheese on it. Cover it with the second slice and it is ready to serve.

Nutrition: Protein 42.8g, Fats 43.2g, Calories 701.4, Sugar 6.6g, Carbohydrates 35.7g, Cholesterol 140.8mg.

Asian Chicken Salad

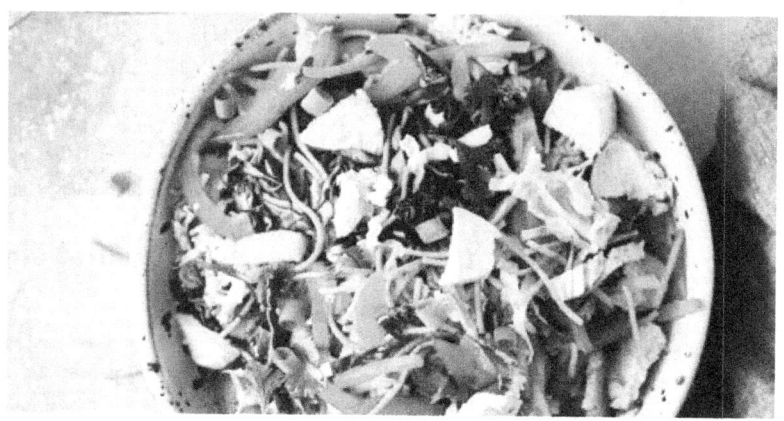

*Preparation time: 20 minutes | **Cooking time**: 10 minutes | **Servings**: 6*

Ingredients:
- 1 thinly sliced red bell pepper
- 1 peeled and sliced carrot
- 2 thinly sliced chicken breasts
- 1 shredded lettuce
- 1 shredded cabbage
- ½ teaspoon salt and black pepper
- 2 tablespoons chopped basil leaves

- ½ cup toasted almonds
- 2 tablespoons soy sauce
- 2 tablespoons grated sugar
- ¼ cup vegetable oil
- 1 tablespoon vinegar

Directions: Grill the thinly sliced chicken. Take a bowl and add bell pepper, carrot, grilled chicken, lettuce, cabbage, basil, almonds, salt, and pepper. Mix all the ingredients well. Now for dressing mix sauce, sugar, vinegar, and vegetable in a bowl. Pour it over the salad and present it.

Nutrition: Protein 15.1g, Fats 8.1g, Calories 210, Sugar 6g, Carbohydrates 20g, Cholesterol 21mg

Keto Chicken Lettuce Wraps

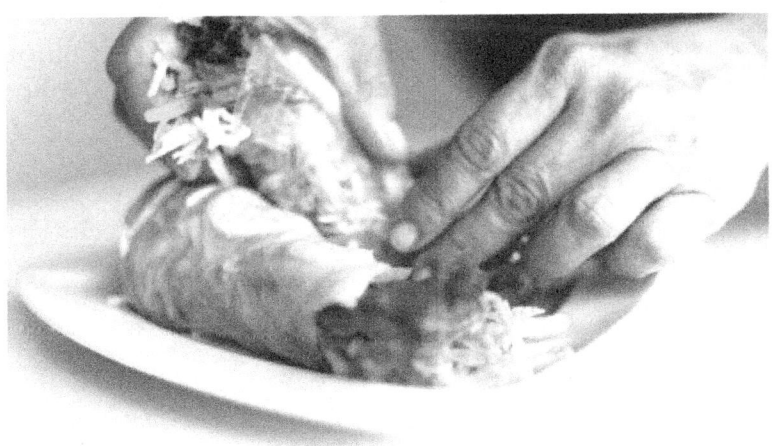

Preparation time: 10 minutes / *Cooking time*: 15 minutes / *Servings*: 12

Ingredients:

- 2 shredded chicken breasts
- 1 cup diced tomatoes
- ½ teaspoon salt
- ½ teaspoon black pepper
- 1 sliced green onion
- 1 diced avocado
- ½ cup grated cheese
- 2 teaspoons lemon juice
- 12 leaves of lettuce

Directions:

In a pan boil the shredded chicken for around 15 minutes. Take a bowl and add all the ingredients leaving lettuce leaves. Add the boiled and shredded chicken in it as well and mix all the ingredients thoroughly. Take lettuce leaves and put a small amount of batter on all the leaves and wrap them. Serve it cold.

Nutrition: Protein 9g, Fats 5g, Calories 93, Carbohydrates 2g, Cholesterol 29mg, Fiber 1g.

Egg And Vegetable Bagel Sandwich

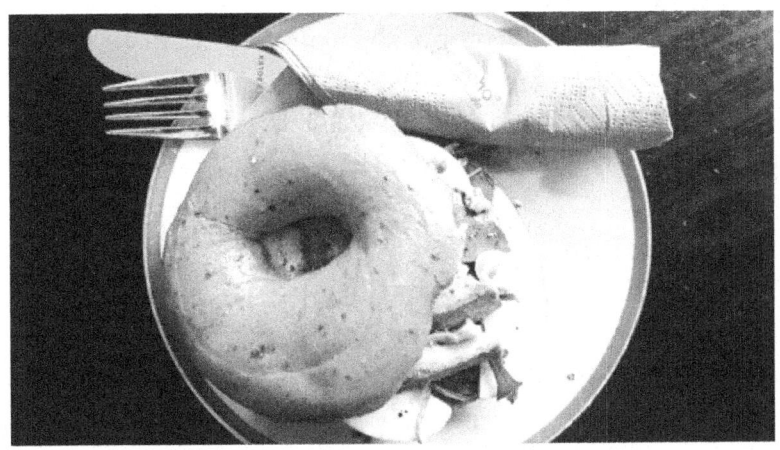

Preparation time: 05 minutes I Cooking time: 05-07 minutes I Servings: 1

Ingredients:
- 1 thin bagel
- 1 tablespoon olive oil
- 2 sliced mushrooms
- ½ sliced avocado
- ½ cup crushed spinach leaves
- 2 eggs whites
- ½ cup cubed tomatoes
- ½ cup diced red pepper
- A pinch of salt
- ½ teaspoon crushed black pepper
- 2 slices of wheat bread

Directions:
Take a pan and toss thin bagel in olive oil. After that in the same pan add oil and sauté the mushrooms, spinach leaves, avocado, red pepper,

tomatoes, and add salt and pepper. Now cook the egg white. Take the bread slices and spread the bagel, eggs, and veggies on it in the form of layers. place the second slice on it and serve it.

Nutrition: Protein 13.1g, Fats 7.2g, Calories 278.6, Carbohydrates 42.1g, Fiber 4.0g.

Chicken Caprese Sandwich

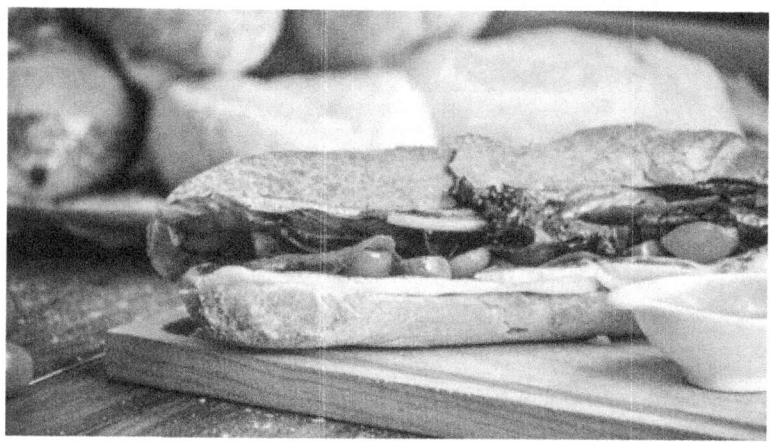

Preparation time: 10 minutes | **Cooking time**: 10 minutes | **Servings**: 4

Ingredients:
- ¼ cup prepared pesto
- 4 boneless chicken halves
- 8 basil leaves
- ¼ cup mayonnaise
- A pinch of salt and black pepper
- 1 sliced tomato
- 1 tablespoon olive oil
- 4 slices mozzarella cheese

- 4 slices of sandwich bread

Directions:
Grill the chicken with seasoning black pepper, salt, and olive oil. Grill the chicken for around 10 minutes. In a bowl mix the mayonnaise and pesto. Toast the bread slices and spread the mixed mayonnaise. Place the grilled chicken, leaves, tomatoes, and mozzarella cheese slice and serve it.

Nutrition: Protein 37g, fats 28g, Calories 542, Carbohydrates 33g, Fiber 1g.

Slow-Cooker Split Pea Soup

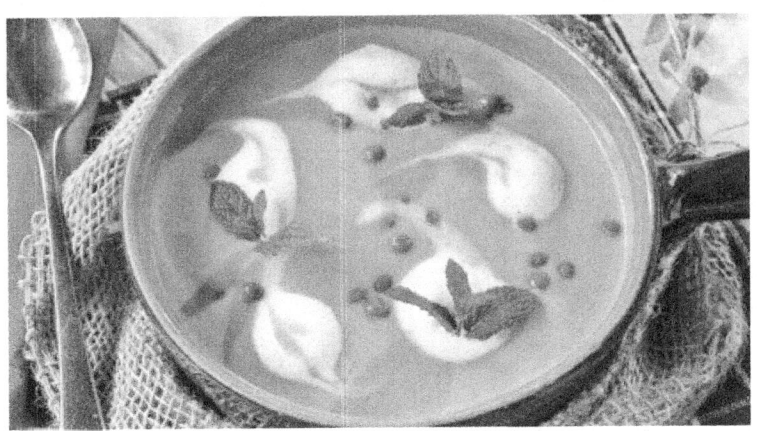

Preparation time: *10-15 minutes* / *Cooking time*: *6-8 hours* / *Servings*: *8*

Ingredients:
- 2 cups fully cooked ham

- 1 chopped large onion
- 1 cup chopped carrots
- 3 minced garlic cloves
- 16 ounces dried split green peas

- 32 ounces chicken broth
- ½ teaspoon dried thyme
- ½ teaspoon crushed dried rosemary
- 2 cups of water

Directions:

Take a slow cooker and add all the ingredients in it. Combine and mix them well. Cover the slow cooker and cook it on a medium flame for 6 to 8 hours. Cook until peas become soft. If you are using the uncooked ham it will take 10 hours to cook.

Nutrition: Protein 23g, Fats 2g, Calories 260, Sugar 7g, Carbohydrates 39g, Cholesterol 21mg.

Cobb Egg Salad

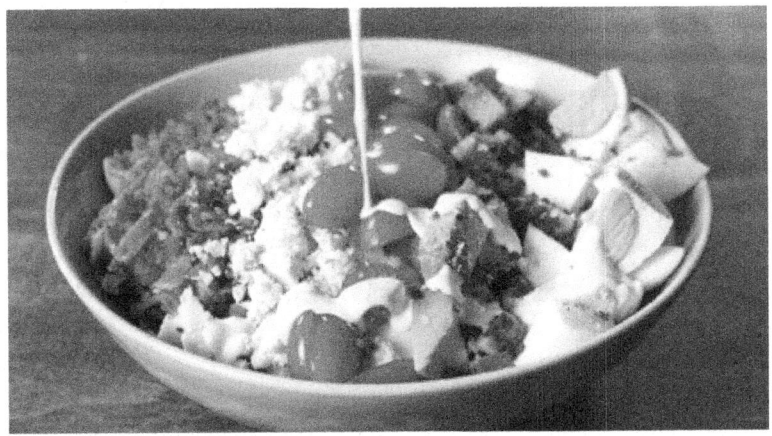

Preparation time: 10 minutes / *Chilling time*: 5 minutes / *Servings*: 6

Ingredients:
- 3 tablespoons yogurt
- 8 hard-boiled eggs
- 3 tablespoons mayonnaise

- a pinch of crushed black pepper
- 2 tablespoons red wine vinegar
- a pinch of salt
- 8 strips of cooked bacon
- ½ cup finely grated cheese
- 1 thinly sliced avocado2 tablespoons crushed chives
- ½ cup cherry and tomatoes (for garnishing)

Directions:
Take a bowl and smashed the boiled eggs. Now add all the ingredients in the same bowl expect cherry

and tomatoes. Mix all the ingredients until they combine well. Put it in the refrigerator for 5 minutes so that all the ingredients set well. Serve it after garnishing it with cherry and tomatoes.

Nutrition: Protein 13g, Fats 5g, Calories 235, Sugar 2g, Carbohydrates 9g, Cholesterol 195mg, Fiber 3g.

Chicken Cheese Sandwich

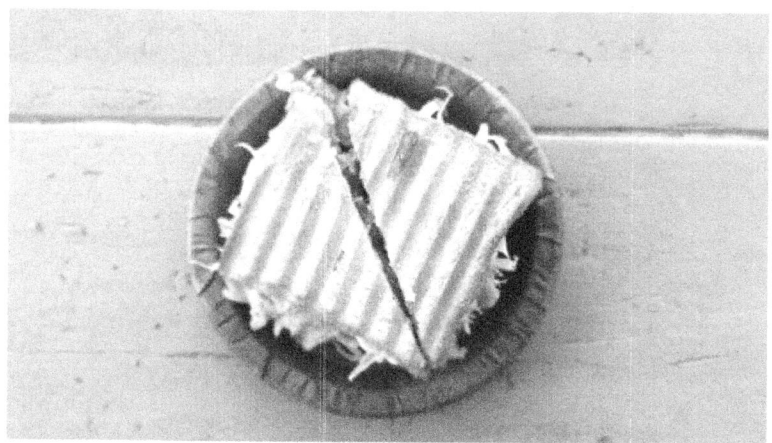

*Preparation time: 10 minutes I **Cooking time**: 5 minutes I **Servings**: 4*

Ingredients:
- 4 tablespoons mayonnaise
- 1 ½ cups boiled and shredded chicken
- ½ cup thinly sliced cucumber

- ½ cup red capsicum
- ½ teaspoon crushed black pepper

- a pinch of salt

- ½ teaspoon crushed white pepper

- ½ cup sweet corn
- ½ cup finely grated cheese

- 2 tablespoons butter
- 8-10 slices of sandwich bread

Directions:
Take a bowl and add all the ingredients in it except bread, butter, and cheese. Combine the ingredients properly. Now take the sandwich bread slices and cut its hard sides. Apply some butter on the one side of all the slices and toast them from both sides. Now add cheese and prepared mixture on it. And put the second slice on it. Cut it in the triangular shape and serve it.

Nutrition: Protein 8g, Fats 29g, Calories 369, Sugar 2g, Carbohydrates 16g, Cholesterol 35mg, Fiber 1g.

Charred Shrimp And Avocado

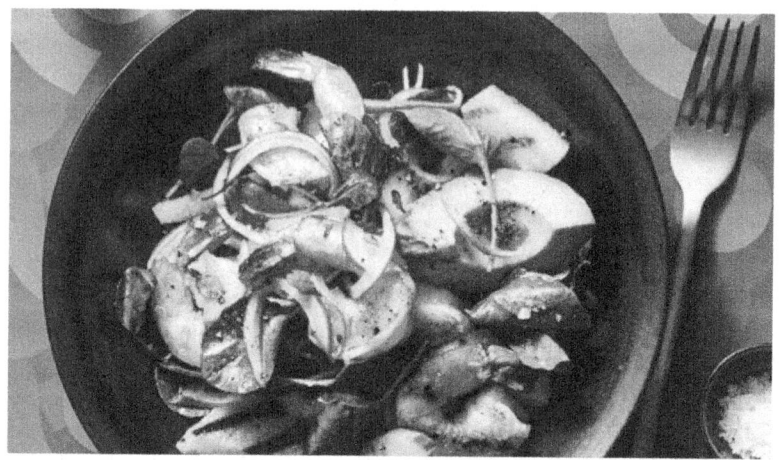

Preparation time: *10 minutes* | **Cooking time**: *15 minutes* | **Servings**: *4*

Ingredients:
- 5 tablespoons olive oil
- 2 ½ lb. peeled large shrimp
- ½ teaspoon salt
- 1 cup peeled and cubed cut pineapple
- ½ cup thinly sliced onion
- 1 avocado
- 2 tablespoons lemon juice
- ½ cup finely peeled and cut cucumber
- ½ finely chopped upland watercress
- ½ teaspoon crushed
- black pepper

Directions:

Take a pan and toss shrimp in oil, salt, and pepper. Grill pineapple after brushing oil on both sides. Grill shrimp and pineapple for 3 minutes each side. Take another bowl and put all the remaining ingredients and mix them well. Now add the toasted shrimp and pineapple in it and present it.

Nutrition: Protein 35g, fats 23.5g, Calories 420, Carbohydrates 20g, Fiber 4g.

Grilled Steak Tortilla

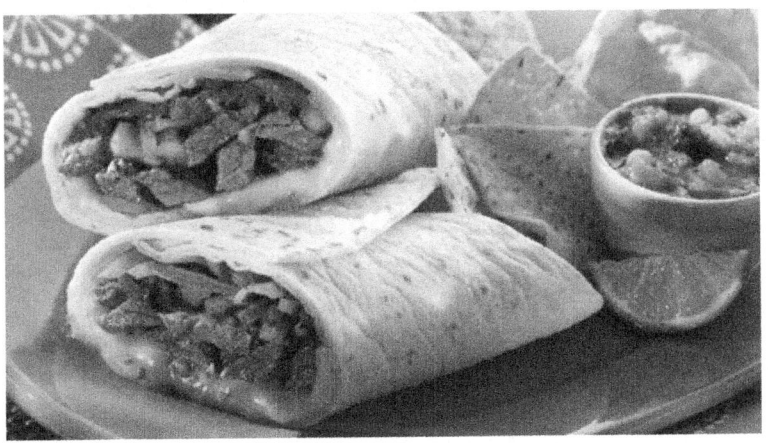

Preparation time: 10 minutes I Cooking time: 20 minutes I Servings: 4

Ingredients:
- 1 cup cubed cut tomatoes
- 1 cup brisket
- 1 teaspoon red chili powder
- 2 sliced cut spring onions
- 1 cup coriander
- 2 tablespoons lemon juice
- 1 sliced cut jalapeno
- 1 bunch of rocket
- 4 quarter cut flour tortillas

- 1 teaspoon salt

Directions:
Grill the brisket with salt and paper for around 5 minutes. Mix the rest of the ingredients except tortillas. Cut the slices of the grilled brisket and combine it in the mixture. Serve it with flour tortillas.

Nutrition: Protein 41g, fats 5g, Calories 420, Carbohydrates 9g, Fiber 3g.

Dinner Recipes

One-Pot Beef With Broccoli

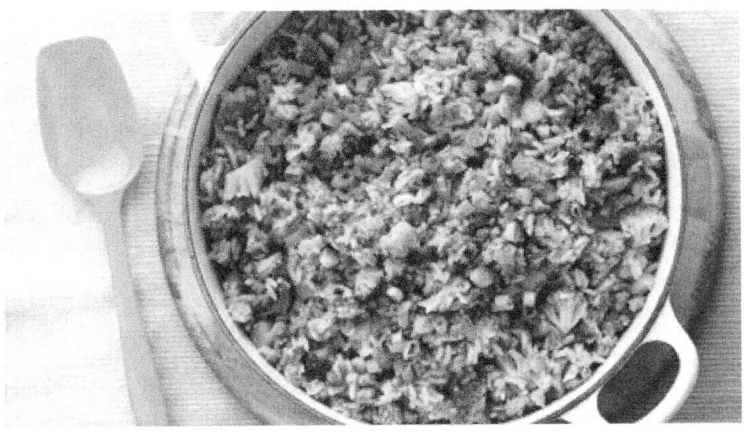

***Preparation time**: 10 minutes | **Cooking time**: 10 minutes | **Servings**: 5*

Ingredients:
- 1½ cups chopped and cooked broccoli
- 1lb minced beef
- 3 cups cooked cold white rice
- 1 bunch chopped green onion
- ½ cup diced chopped white onion
- 1 cup teriyaki marinade and sauce
- A pinch of salt

Directions:

Take a nonstick pan with oil and cook beef over medium flame. Add salt in it and stir it continuously. Cook it for 5 to 7 minutes. Add onions in it and cook for one minute now add rice and teriyaki and sauce and cook for 2 minutes. Add broccoli in it and mix well. its ready to present.

Nutrition: Protein 28g, Fats 35g, Calories 460, Carbohydrates 7g, Fiber 1g.

Sheet Pan Sausages & Veggies

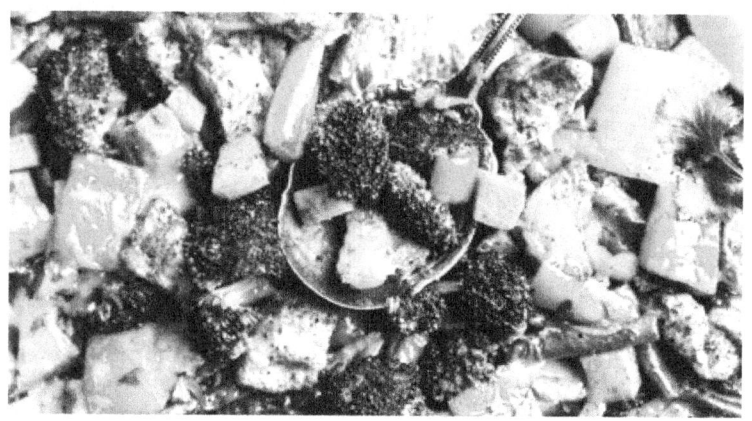

Preparation time: 10 minutes / *Cooking time:* 20 minutes / *Servings: 4*

Ingredients:
- 1 diced red bell pepper
- 16 ounces smoked sausage
- 1 cup cubed radish
- ½ minced onion
- 1 teaspoon Italian seasoning
- 1 teaspoon salt
- 1 tablespoon halved parsley

- ½ teaspoon cracked pepper
- 2 tablespoons avocado oil
- 12 ounces florets broccoli

Directions:
Prepare a baking dish with liner and preheat the oven at 400F. Take a bowl and add all the ingredients except broccoli in it and mix them well. On the prepared baking dish spread the mixture in the single layer. Bake it for around 20 minutes in the preheated oven. Stir it once while baking. Sprinkle parsley on it and serve.

Nutrition: Protein 16g, Fats 39g, Calories 460, Carbohydrates 11g, Fiber 4g.

Loaded Sheet Pan Nachos

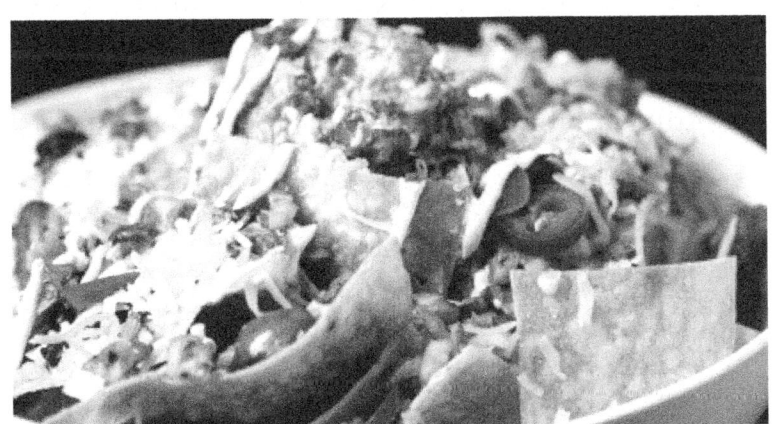

Preparation time: *15 minutes I Cooking time:* *10 minutes I Servings: 8*

Ingredients:

- 1 pound ground beef
- 12 ounces tortilla chips
- 1 tablespoon olive oil
- 2 chopped garlic cloves
- 1.25-ounce taco seasoning
- 1 cup roasted corn kernels
- 1 cup shredded cheddar cheese
- ½ cup grated Jack cheese
- 2 tablespoons sour cream
- 2 tablespoons chopped cilantro leaves
- 1 diced tomato
- 1 thinly sliced jalapeno

Directions:

Preheat the oven at 400F and prepare a baking dish with a baking sheet. Take a skillet with olive oil over the medium flame. Cook beef with garlic and cook it for 5 minutes. Add taco seasoning o it. In the baking dish place the chips in a single layer and spread beef mixture on it. Add beans, cheese, and corn on it and bake for 5 minutes. Topped it with remaining ingredients and serve it immediately.

Nutrition: Protein 24.3g, Fats 25.8g, Calories 493, Carbohydrates 44.1g, Fiber 7g.

Lemon & Garlic Salmon With Asparagus

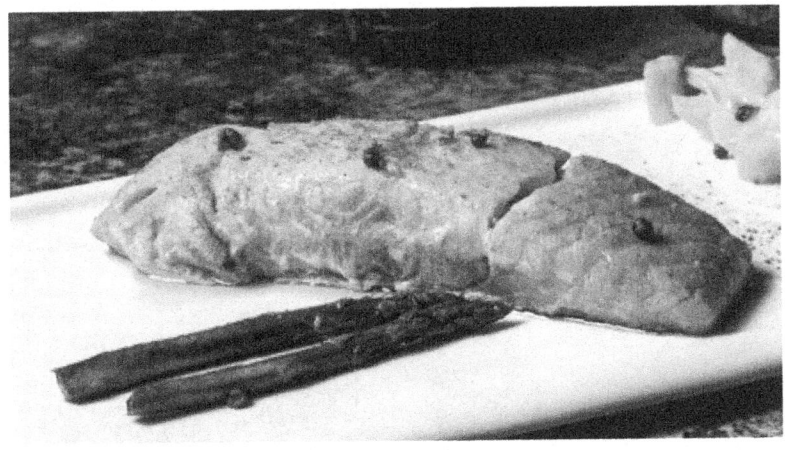

Preparation time: *05 minutes I* **Cooking time**: *10 minutes I* **Servings**: *3*

Ingredients:
- 1 tablespoon salted butter
- 2 chopped garlic cloves
- 1 tablespoon olive oil

- 1 trimmed bunch of asparagus
- 1 pound fillet cut salmon
- ½ tablespoon lemon juice
- ½ teaspoon salt and black pepper

Directions:
Heat the butter and olive oil in a skillet. Add asparagus and salmon in it and season with pepper and salt. Cook it for around 3 to 4 minutes on each side. Add garlic and lemon juice and cook for 1 to

2 minutes more. Convert it into the serving dish and serve.

Nutrition: Protein 32.8g, Fats 28.8g, Calories 409, Carbohydrates 4.6g, Cholesterol 93.3mg.

Slow Cooker BBQ Chicken

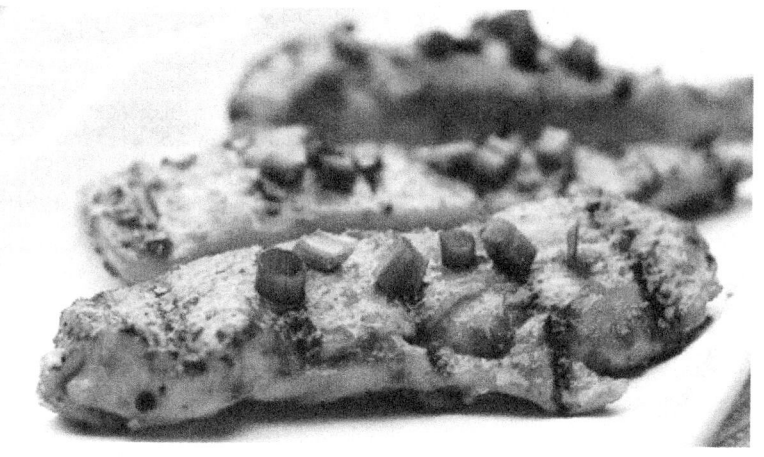

Preparation time: 5 minutes / *Cooking time:* 4 hours / *Servings:* 4

Ingredients:
- 4 boneless chicken breasts
- ½ chopped onion
- 1 tablespoon soy sauce
- 1½ cups BBQ sauce
- 1 tablespoon olive oil
- 2 tablespoons brown sugar

Directions:

In a slow cooker add all the ingredients and mix them well. Coat the chicken in sauce mixture thoroughly. Cover and cook it on medium heat for 4 hours. Now remove the chicken in a trey and shred it with the help of forks. Serve it with some BBQ sauce topping.

Nutrition: Protein 23.1g, Fats 2.8g, Calories 364, Carbohydrates 59.9g.

Crispy Cauliflower Tacos

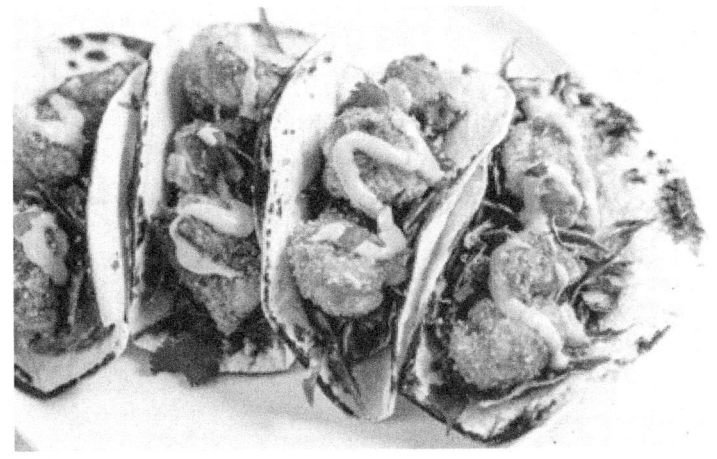

Preparation time: 15 minutes I Cooking time: 30 minutes I Servings: 12

Ingredients:
- ¾ cup chickpea flour
- ¾ cup almond milk
- 3 tablespoons taco seasoning
- 1 ½ cup cornmeal

- 1 cauliflower
- 3 cups grated cabbage
- 12 sugar free tortillas
- 2 tablespoons yeast
- ½ teaspoon salt and pepper

Directions:

Cut the cauliflower in thick pieces. Take a bowl and mix the flour and almond milk in it and leave it for few minutes. In another bowl mix yeast, taco, salt and pepper, and cornmeal. Now dip each piece of cauliflower in the flour and yeast mixture one by one. Set this cauliflower on the baking sheet and put it in the preheated oven with 400F temperature for 25 to 30 minutes. Now place the pieces of backed cauliflower in the tortillas and add cabbage on it. And it's ready to serve.

Nutrition: Protein 10g, Fats 5g, Calories 230, Carbohydrates 37g, Fiber 9g.

Chicken Scampi Pasta

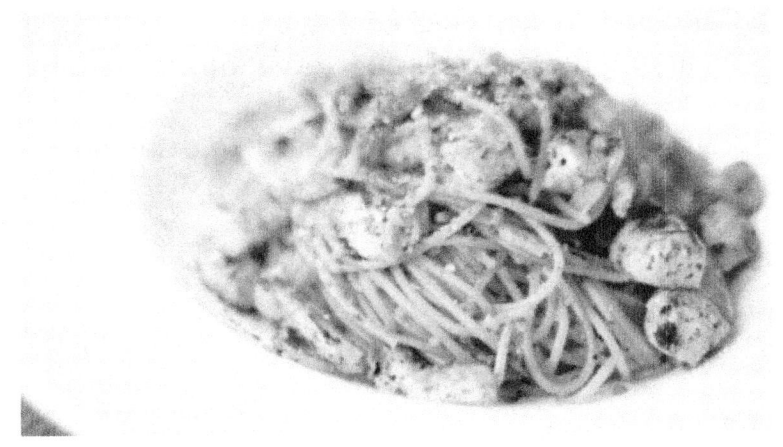

Preparation time: 10 minutes / **Cooking time**: 10 minutes / **Servings**: 6

Ingredients:
- 2 cups boiled pasta
- 3 sliced chicken breasts
- 1 finely sliced bell pepper
- 1 tablespoon Italian seasoning
- ½ sliced cut onion
- 2 cups chicken broth
- 1 minced garlic clove
- ½ teaspoon salt
- ½ teaspoon black pepper
- 1 cup sheared cheese

Directions:
Take a skillet and place the sliced chicken breast in it. Cook it over medium-high flame until its color started to change. Add onion and bell peppers in it and cook for more 2 to 3 minutes. Add broth in it and when it starts simmering reduce the heat and cover it with the lid. Take a dish with boiled pasta

and add cooked chicken and cheese on it. Sprinkle salt and pepper on it and serve it immediately.

Nutrition: Protein 29g, fats 7g, Calories 435, Carbohydrates 60g, Fiber 3g.

Chicken Steak With Stuffed Potatoes

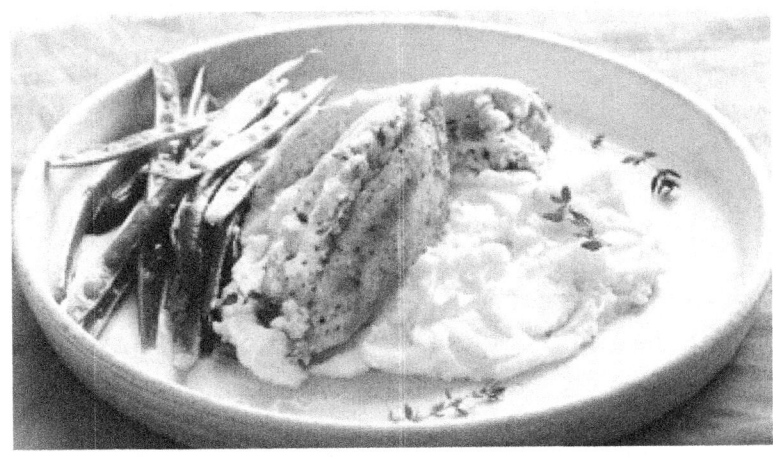

Preparation time: 25 minutes / **Cooking time**: 45 minutes / **Servings**: 4

Ingredients:

- 2 potatoes
- 4 chicken breasts
- ½ teaspoon salt
- 1 tablespoon olive oil
- ½ teaspoon crushed black pepper
- 1 tablespoon butter
- 1 minced garlic clove
- ½ teaspoon salt
- ½ tablespoon lemon juice
- 2 tablespoon ginger and garlic paste
- ½ tablespoon red chilly
- ¼ teaspoon cinnamon powder

Directions:

Peel and cut the potatoes. Boil them on a medium flame for around 20 minutes. Mash these boiled potatoes and mix milk, butter, salt, and black pepper in it. Put it aside. Take the chicken breasts and make a pocket in it by cutting it from the middle. Take a bowl add garlic and ginger paste, lemon juice, red pepper, salt, cinnamon powder in it and mix it well. Marinate the chicken with the mixture and leave it for at least 15 minutes. Stuffed the potato mixture in the chicken breast. Now take a grill pan and cook the chicken stakes for at least 10 minutes. Then low down the flame and cover the pan and cook for more 5 minutes. Take out on the serving plate and serve it.

Nutrition: Protein 19g, Fats 12g, Calories 370, Carbohydrates 69g, Fiber 7g.

Buffalo Chicken Enchiladas

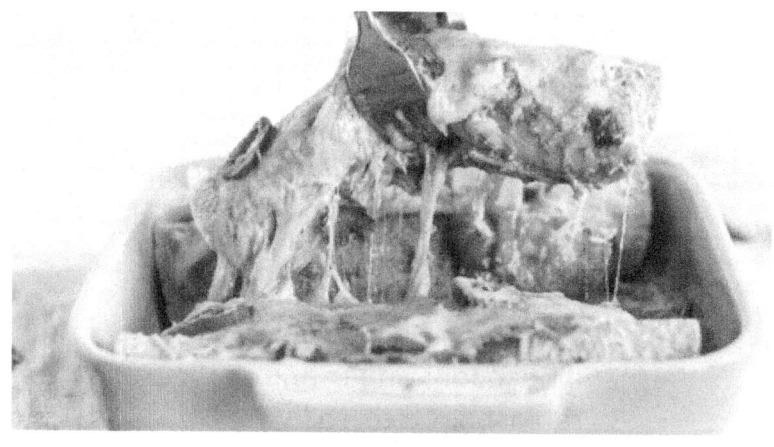

Preparation time: 10 minutes I *Cooking time:* 20 minutes I *Servings:* 4

Ingredients:
- ½ teaspoon seasoning

- 1 boiled and shredded chicken breast
- ½ cup buffalo sauce

- ½ cup enchilada sauce
- ½ cup cubed cut tomatoes
- 5 flour tortillas
- 1 cup shredded cheese
- ½ teaspoon crushed green chilies

Directions:
Prepare the baking dish with a baking sheet and add the half enchilada sauce in it. Preheat the oven at the 350F temperature. Take a bowl and mix the chicken, buffalo sauce, remaining enchilada sauce, tomatoes and green chilly in it and combine well. Take the tortillas and pour chicken mixture in its middle and add cheese on its top. Now fold it from two sides on the filling portion. Set them in the baking dish and add cheese and sauces on its top. Now bake it in the preheated oven for around 20 minutes.

Nutrition: Protein 15g, Fats 3g, Calories 191, Carbohydrates 22g, Fiber 1g, Cholesterol 36mg.

Hot Sausages Cast-Iron Skillet Pan Pizza

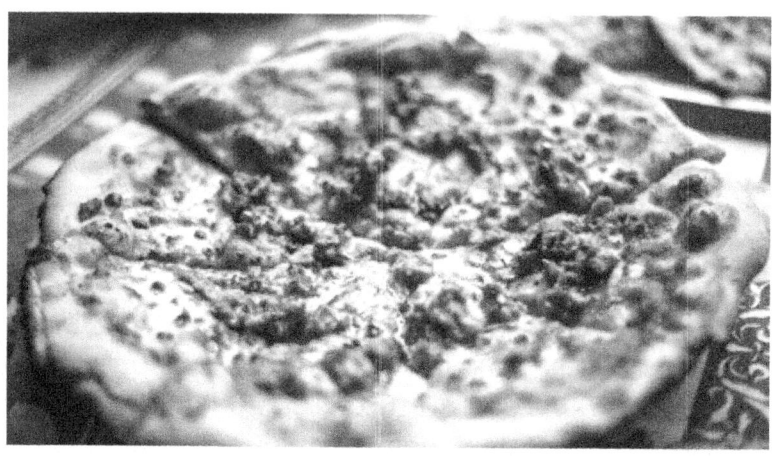

Preparation time: *15 minutes I* ***Cooking time:*** *30 minutes I **Servings:** 4*

Ingredients:
- 2 tablespoons tomato paste
- 1 cup cubed tomatoes
- A pinch of salt and black pepper
- a pinch of sugar
- ¼ teaspoon oregano
- 1 minced garlic clove
- 6-7 leaves of basil
- 1 pound pizza dough
- ¼ cup oil
- ½ pound diced hot sausage
- 3 cups grated cheese

Directions:

In a blender add tomato paste, garlic, oregano, basil, sugar, and salt and blend it well. Take a greased skillet and stretch the dough in the even round shape. Take a pan with oil and cook the sausages until it changes its color. Now take the pan and set the pizza dough in it. Now brush oil on the dough and add the blended sauce on it. Add cooked sausages, and cheese. Now cook it on the medium-low flame for around 3 minutes. Transfer it from skillet to the baking dish. And bake it in the preheated oven at the 475F temperature for around 15 minutes.

Nutrition: Protein 36g, Fats 3g, Calories 390, Carbohydrates 29g, Fiber 5g.

Delicious Snacks Recipes

Potato Lollipop

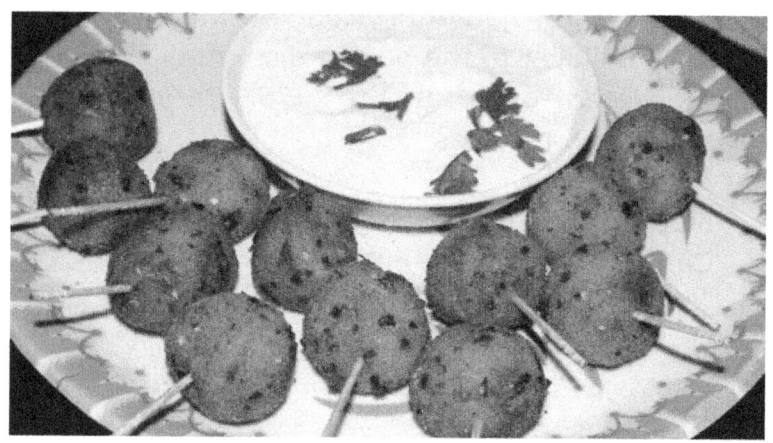

Preparation time: 15 minutes / **Cooking time**: 15 minutes / **Servings**: 3

Ingredients:

- 2 large boiled and peeled potatoes

- 2 chopped green chilies
- 2 slices of bread
- 1 boiled and peeled carrot
- ½ teaspoon ginger paste
- 2 teaspoons corn flour
- ½ teaspoon cumin powder

- 2 cups oil
- ½ teaspoon salt
- ½ teaspoon chaat masala powder

Directions:

In a bowl mash the boiled potatoes and add carrots, ginger, green chilies, chaat masala, cumin powder, and salt in it and mix all the ingredients properly. Soak the slices of bread in water for 3 minutes and squeeze the water properly. Add in the potato mixture and add corn flour too. Mix all the ingredients and make small balls with this dough. Shallow fry these balls properly and insert a lollipop stick in it and serve.

Nutrition: Protein 2g, Fats 3g, Calories 187, Carbohydrates 12g, Fiber 1g, Cholesterol 1mg.

Potato Cheese Balls

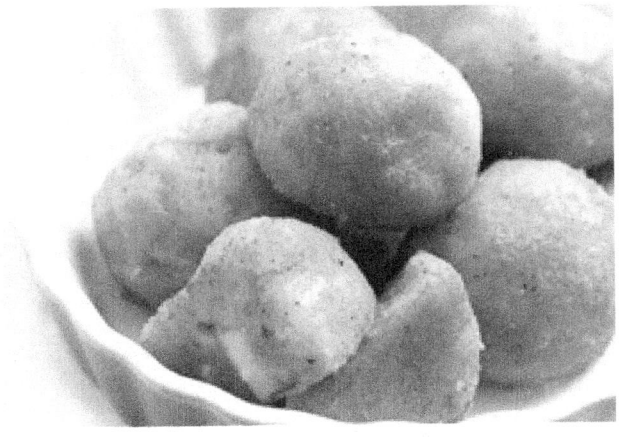

Preparation time: 15 minutes I *Cooking time:* 10 minutes I *Servings:* 10

Ingredients:

- 2 ½ cups boiled mashed potatoes
- ½ cup cheddar cheese
- ½ teaspoon salt
- ½ teaspoon white pepper
- 1 cup breadcrumbs
- 2 lightly beaten eggs
- 1 cup flour
- 1 cup vegetable oil

Directions:
Take a bowl and add mashed potatoes, salt, and white pepper mix it well. Now make balls of it by adding small cheese slice in its middle. Now coat it in the flour, egg, and breadcrumbs in a sequence. Shallow fry them in the vegetable oil on the medium heat. Serve them immediately.

Nutrition: Fats 4g, Calories 110, Carbohydrates 15g, Cholesterol 24mg.

Crispy Pepperoni Chips

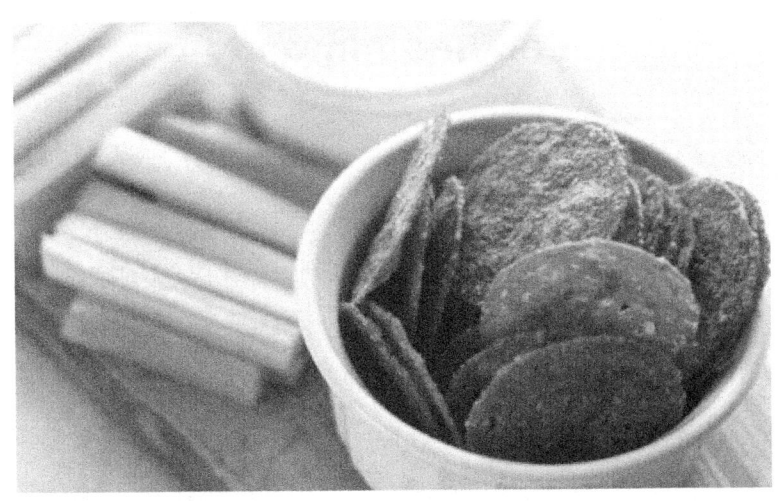

Preparation time: 05 minutes / **Cooking time**: 15 minutes / **Servings**: 4

Ingredients:
- 6 ounces thinly sliced pepperoni

Directions:
Preheat the oven at the 425 degrees F temperature. Prepare a baking dish with liner. Spread the pepperoni slices on baking dish in a single layer. Bake it in the preheated oven for around 10 minutes. Take out the pan from the oven and with the help of a soaking sheet or towel soak the excess grease from the pepperoni. Put the pan in the oven again for around 4 to 5 minutes until pepperoni slices become crispy.

Nutrition: Fats 14g, Calories 150, Carbohydrates 1g, Cholesterol 30mg, Protein 5g

Candied Almonds

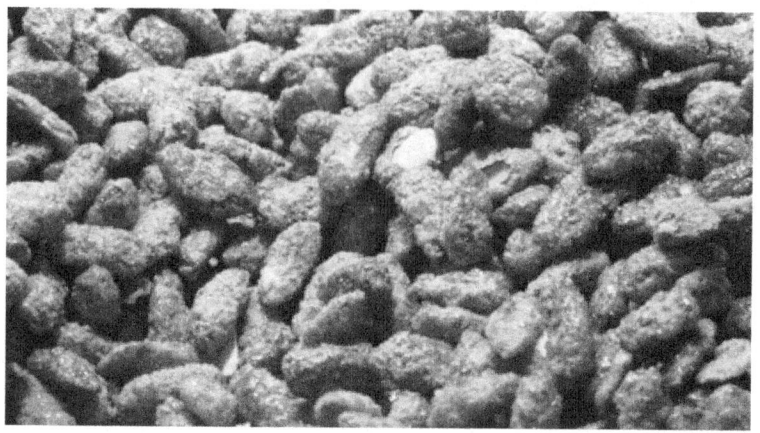

Preparation time: 05 minutes / **Cooking time:** 15 minutes / **Servings:** 08

Ingredients:
- 1 cup white sugar
- ½ cup water
- 2 cups almonds
- 1 tablespoon ground cinnamon

Directions:
In a pan add water, cinnamon, and sugar and put it on the medium flame. When it starts boiling add almonds in it. Cook it until the water evaporates and the mixture transformed in the form of a syrup or coating around the almonds. Now dish out the coated almond and leave them to cool for 15 minutes. Now it is ready to present.

Nutrition: Fats 18g, Calories 304, Carbohydrates 32.7g, Protein 7.6g.

Wheat Crackers

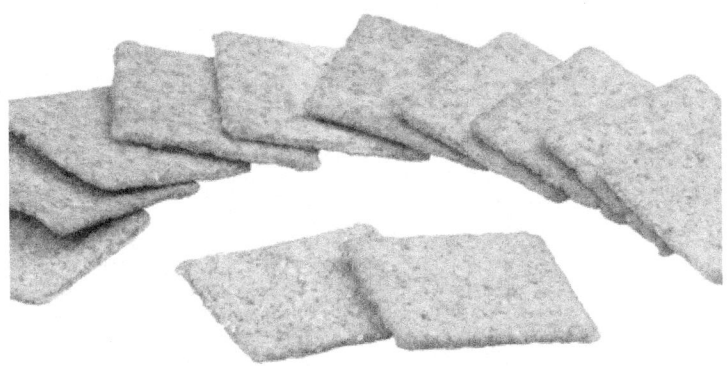

Preparation time: 10 minutes / **Cooking time**: 20 minutes / **Servings**: 32

Ingredients:

- 1 ½ cups all-purpose flour
- 1 ¾ cups whole wheat flour
- 1/3 cup vegetable oil
- ¾ teaspoon salt
- 1 cup of water

Directions:

In a bowl add all the ingredients and mix them until it gets the form of a dough. Preheat the oven at 350F temperature. Roll out the prepared dough on a light surface with flour in a thinner layer. It should be thinner than 1/8 inch. Now place it in the ungreased baking dish. With the help of knife mark squares and with the help of fork prick each piece of cracker. Sprinkle a pinch of salt and bake it for 20 minutes or until it becomes crispy.

Nutrition: Fats 2.5g, Calories 64, Carbohydrates 9.2g, Protein 1.5g.

Yummy Snacks Option

Cranberry Nut Granola Bar

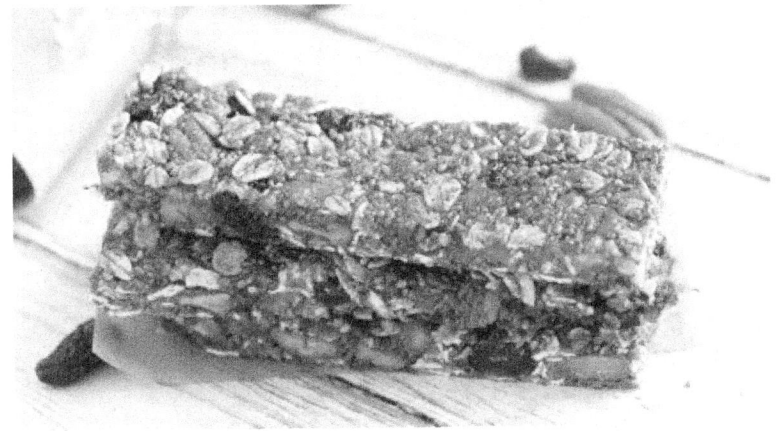

Preparation time: 10 minutes / Cooking time: 20 minutes / Servings: 24

Ingredients:
- ½ cup slivered almonds
- 1 cup mix nuts
- 2 cups oats
- ½ cup hulled pumpkin seeds
- 1 cup condensed milk
- 1 cup cranberries

Directions:
In a mixing bowl mix all the ingredients thoroughly. Preheat the oven at the temperature of 350F. Prepare a baking dish with greased baking liner on

all sides. Spread it into the baking dish in a thick layer evenly. Bake it in for around 20 to 25 minutes. Let it be cool for 5 minutes and cut it in the form of bars with a sharp knife and serve it.

Nutrition: Fats 7.5g, Calories 169, Carbohydrates 22.3g, Protein 4.8g.

Bacon Avocado Fries

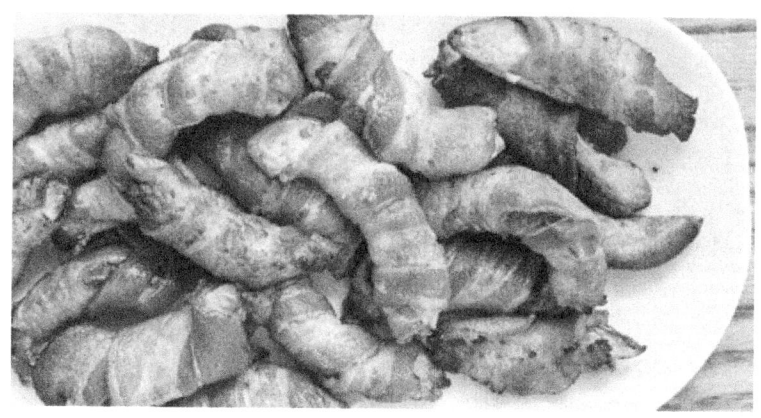

Preparation time: 10 minutes I *Chilling time*: 15 minutes I *Servings*: 20

Ingredients:
- 3 thinly sliced avocados
- 20 thin strips bacon
- ¼ cup ranch dressing (optional)

Directions:

Prepare a baking dish with a greased baking sheet. Set the oven at 425F temperature to preheat. Take a thin slice of avocado and wrap it in the bacon slice properly. Wrap all the avocado slices in the bacon slices. Place them in the prepared baking dish and bake for around 15 minutes or until it becomes crispy. Now pour ranch dressing on it if you want to.

Nutrition: Fats 65.9g, Calories 693, Carbohydrates 10.9g, Protein 16.3g.

Jalapeno Popper Crisps

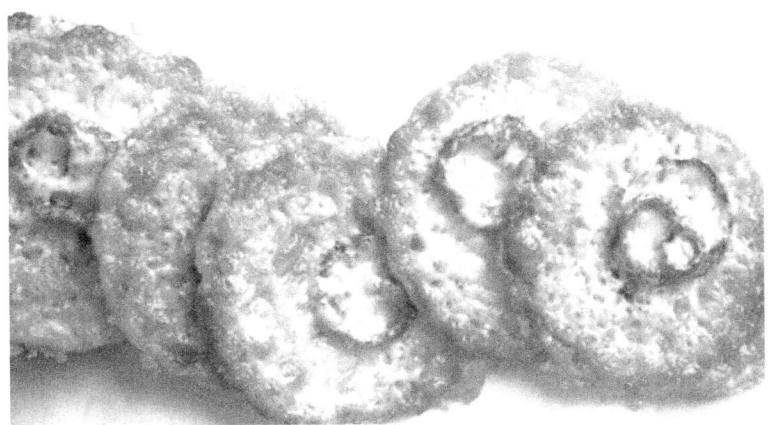

Preparation time: 10 minutes / *Cooking time:* 15 minutes / *Servings:* 8

Ingredients:
- 1 cup grated parmesan
- ½ cup grated cheddar cheese
- ½ teaspoon crushed black pepper
- 1 thinly sliced jalapeno

- 4 slices bacon

Directions:
Preheat the oven at the 375F. In a nonstick skillet cook the bacon for around 8 minutes. Drain the grease with the help of a paper towel and chop it. In the lined baking dish carefully spread 1 tablespoon parmesan. Add 1 tablespoon cheddar cheese on its top and add a jalapeno slice on it. Now carefully pats with and sprinkle pepper on it. Make such small circles with the same process in the whole tray with some distance. Bake it for 12 minutes and serve it when it slightly cooled down.

Nutrition: Fats 12g, Calories 153, Cholesterol 39mg, Protein 9g.

Peanut Butter Protein Balls

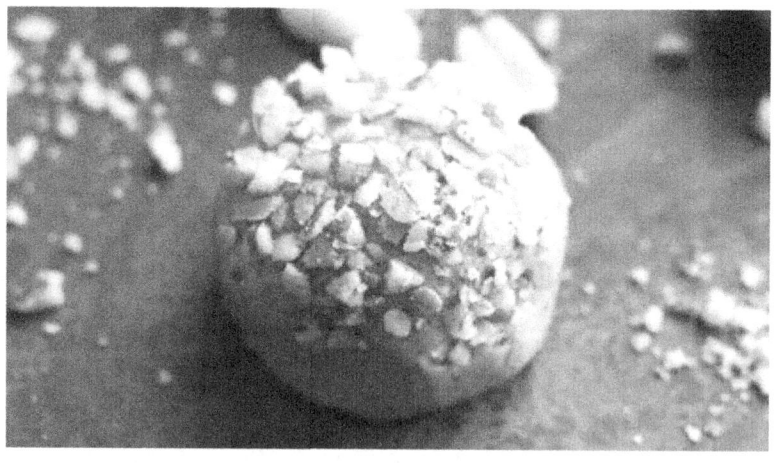

Preparation time: 10 minutes I *Chilling time:* 15 minutes I *Servings:* 15

Ingredients:

- 1 cup unsalted peanut butter
- ½ teaspoon vanilla extract
- 2 teaspoon brown sugar
- 1½ scoops vanilla protein powder
- 20 unsalted raw peanuts
- 1 teaspoon cinnamon

Directions:

Blend the raw peanuts in a blunder and when they become crumbly transfer it to a plate. Take a bowl and add all the ingredients except blended peanuts. Mix them properly. Make the balls with the batter and roll them in the peanut crumble. Set them in a dish and refrigerate it for 15 minutes.

Nutrition: Fats 9.6g, Calories 126, Carbohydrates 4.7g, Protein 7.6g, Sugar 0.7g.

Veggies Cheese Rolls

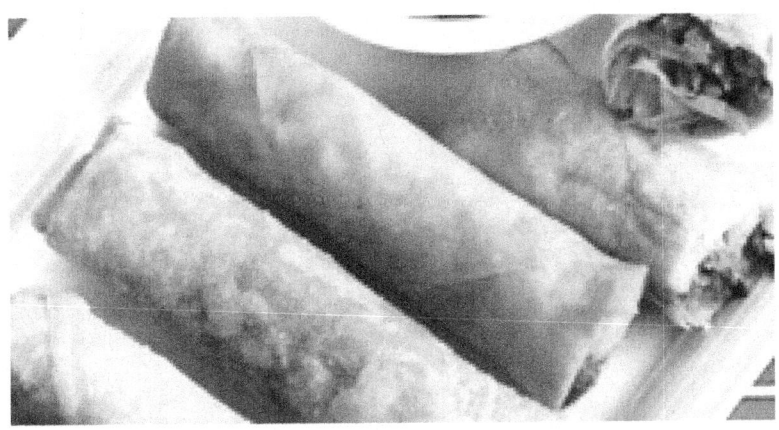

Preparation time: 15 minutes / ***Cooking time:*** 15 minutes / ***Servings:*** 4

Ingredients:
- 1 chopped onion
- 1 chopped tomato
- 1 cup shattered cabbage
- 3 chopped florets broccoli
- 4 tortillas
- ¼ cup coriander leaves
- 2 cups shattered cheese
- 1 beaten egg

Directions:
In a pan sauté the onion, tomato, cabbage, broccoli, coriander leaves for 2 to 3 minutes. In the end, add cheese on it and remove it from the stove. Mix all the ingredients well. Now take the tortillas and add some prepared mixture in it and roll it nicely. Close its sides with beaten egg. Place it in the prepared baking tray with the baking paper. Bake it in the preheated oven with 180C temperature for 20 minutes.

Nutrition: Fats 26g, Calories 391, Carbohydrates 27g, Protein 12g, Sugar 6g.

Strawberry Smoothie

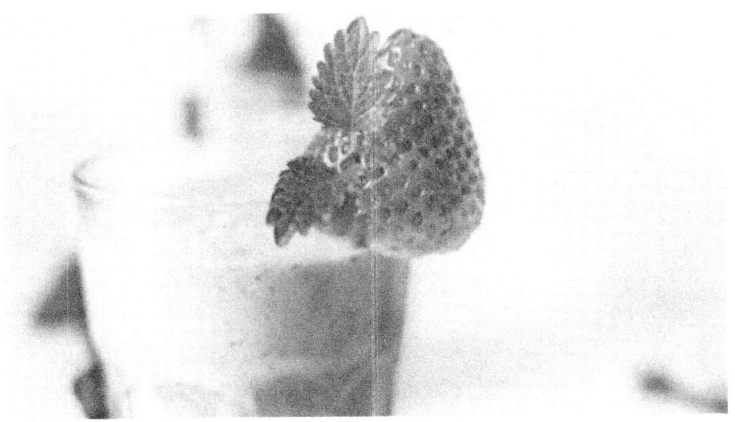

Preparation time*: 5 minutes I **Chilling time***: 30 minutes I **Servings***: 2*

Ingredients:
- 1 cup low-fat milk
- 1 cup frozen strawberries
- 1 tablespoon peanut butter
- 1 teaspoon vanilla extract
- ¼ cup low-fat yogurt

Directions:
Take a high power blender. Put all the ingredients including butter, milk, yogurt, honey, vanilla extract, and strawberries in the blender and blend it until every ingredient merged well. Put it in the glass and leave it to chill for 30 minutes. You can take it immediately as well by adding ice cubes in it.

Nutrition: Protein 6g, Fats 3g, Calories 130, Carbohydrates 15g, Fiber 3g, Cholesterol 1mg.

Caramel Popcorn

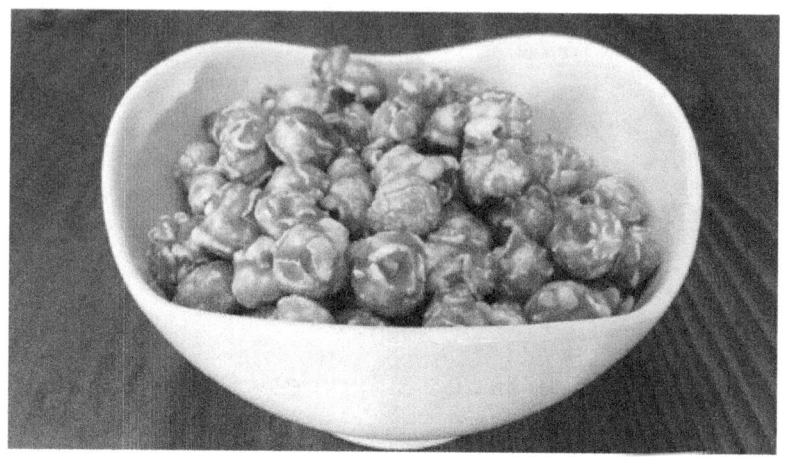

Preparation time: 10 minutes / **Cooking time**:
10 minutes / **Servings**: 10

Ingredients:
- 1 cup butter
- 10 cups popped popcorns
- ½ teaspoon salt
- 2 teaspoons vanilla
- 1 cup brown sugar
- ½ teaspoon baking soda

Directions:
Salt the popped popcorns and set aside. Now take a pan and melt the butter on the medium flame. Add sugar in it and stir it thoroughly and continuously. When it starts boiling leave it on the medium flame for the 5 minutes. Put vanilla in it and mix it well and keep it on the stove for 4

minutes. Now add baking soda in it and cook for another minute. Now pour this mixture on the popcorns and mix it gently. Leave it for some time to keep it cool.

Nutrition: Fats 10g, Calories 245, Carbohydrates 38g, Cholesterol 20mg.

Chocolate Chip Cookies

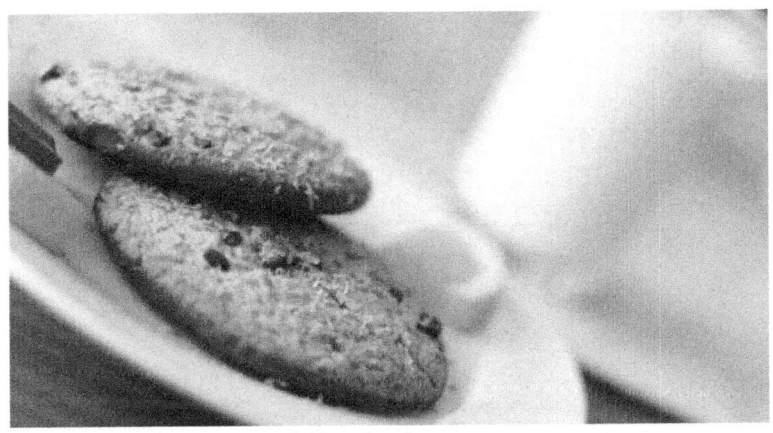

*Preparation time: 10 minutes / **Cooking time:** 8 minutes / **Servings:** 12*

Ingredients:
- 1 cup brown sugar
- 1 cup butter
- 2 teaspoons vanilla extract
- 1 cup white sugar
- 3 cups flour
- 2 large eggs
- 1 teaspoon baking soda
- 1 teaspoon salt
- 2 cups chocolate chips

Directions:
Take a bowl and mix flour, salt, baking powder, and baking soda and set it aside. Add butter and sugar and beat it well. Now add eggs and vanilla in it and beat it well. Mix it in the dry ingredients until it merged well. Add chocolate chips in it. Take a baking dish with baking sheet. Use the scope for making the cookies. Put it in the 375 degrees F preheated oven. And cook it for around 8 to 10 minutes. After 2 minutes remove it in the serving plate.

Nutrition: Fats 12.6g, Calories 263, Carbohydrates 41g, Cholesterol 31.6mg, Protein 2.7g, Sugar 25.5g.

Granola Bars

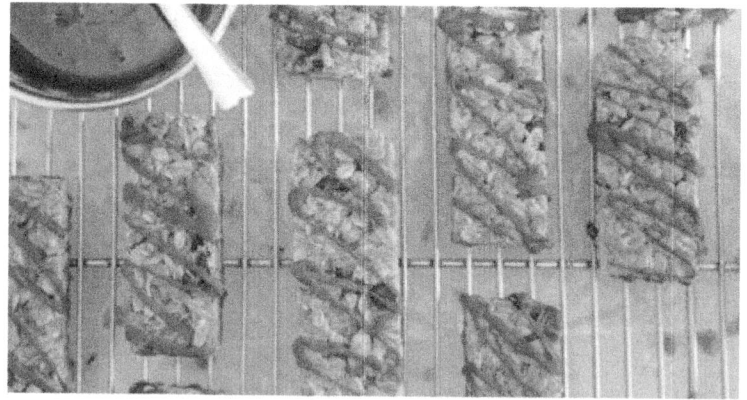

Preparation time: *25 minutes I* *Cooking time:* *25 minutes I* *Servings: 18*
Ingredients:
- 1/3 cup honey

- 2 tablespoons brown sugar
- 6 tablespoons melted butter
- 2 tablespoons maple syrup
- ¼ teaspoon salt
- 1 teaspoon cinnamon powder
- ½ cup shredded coconut
- 3 cups rolled oats
- ½ cup crushed almonds
- 1 ½ cups melted dark chocolate

Directions:
Set the baking tray with baking line and preheat the oven at the 350 degrees F. place a pan on the low medium flame and add honey, butter, cinnamon, maple syrup, and brown sugar. Let it simmer and remove it from the stove when all the ingredients merged well. Now put all the remaining ingredients in it and mix it well. Pour it in the baking tray in an even layer. Bake it in the preheated oven for around 25 to 30 minutes. And cut it in the form of bars.

Nutrition: Fats 13g, Calories 199, Carbohydrates 21g, Cholesterol 10mg, Protein 2g, Sugar 10g.

Nutella Sandwich

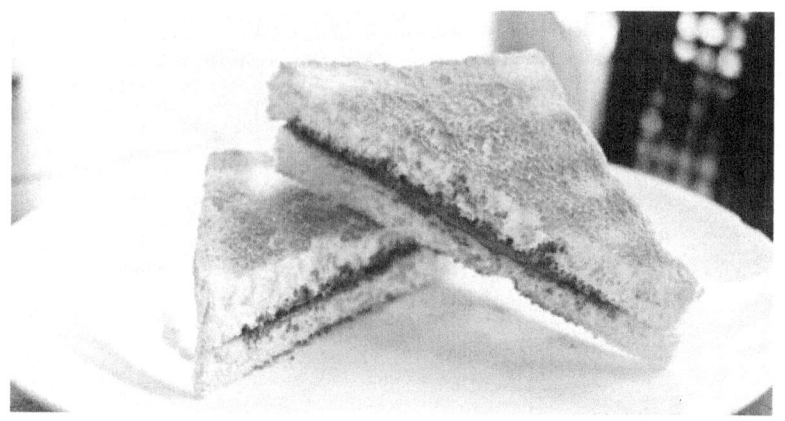

Preparation time: *5 minutes I **Cooking time***: *5 minutes I **Servings***: *3*

Ingredients:
- 6 slices of sandwich bread
- 1 teaspoon butter
- ¾ cup Nutella

Directions:
Take the slices of bread and cut its hard sides. Now apply butter on both sides and grill it for around a minute on each side or until its color changed into golden. Now take the Nutella and apply it on the bread slices. Cut it in the triangular shape and present it. If you are banana lover, you can also use mashed banana in its filling besides Nutella.

Nutrition: Fats 10g, Calories 308, Carbohydrates 46g, Cholesterol 0mg, Protein 6.7g, Sugar 19g.

Oreo Truffles

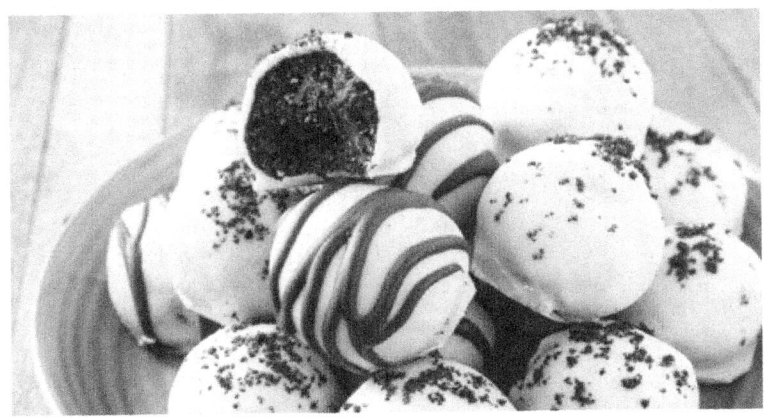

Preparation time*: 05 minutes l **Chilling time***: *1 hour l **Servings**: 12*

Ingredients:
- 8 oz. softened cream cheese
- 14 oz. Oreos
- 2 cups melted white chocolate
- 1 teaspoon vanilla extract
- ½ cup melted the dark chocolate

Directions:
In a blender blend the Oreo cookies to transform it in crumbs. In a bowl mix all the ingredients leaving half white chocolate. Now make small balls of this batter and dip it in the remaining melted white chocolate. Refrigerate it for an hour and serve it.

Nutrition: Fats 6g, Calories 118, Carbohydrates 13g, Protein 1g.

Chocolate Covered Cake Balls

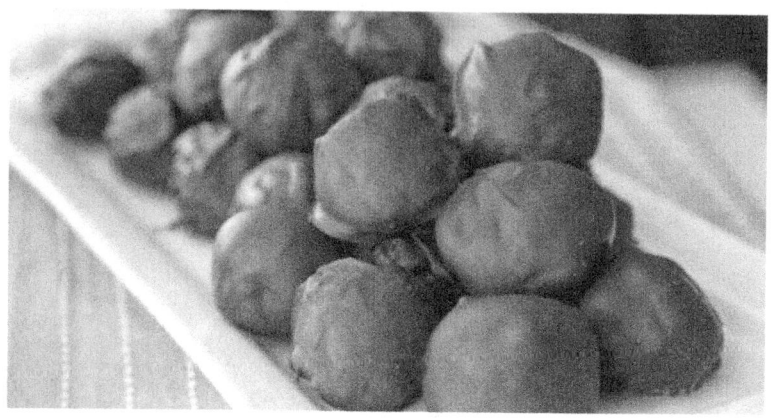

*Preparation time: 10 minutes | **Chilling time**: 1 hour 3' | **Servings**: 25*

Ingredients:
- 18.25 chocolate cake fudge
- 16 oz. prepared chocolate frosting
- 16 oz. dipping chocolate

Directions:
Put the fudge cake into a bowl and crumbled it thoroughly. Add the chocolate frosting in it and mix it well. Make the small balls of this batter and refrigerate it for 20 minutes. Take the balls out and dip them in the dipping chocolate one by one. Now put it back in the refrigerator for one hour and serve it.

Nutrition: Fats 6g, Calories 146, Carbohydrates 22g, sugar 17g.

Pumpkin Cake Roll

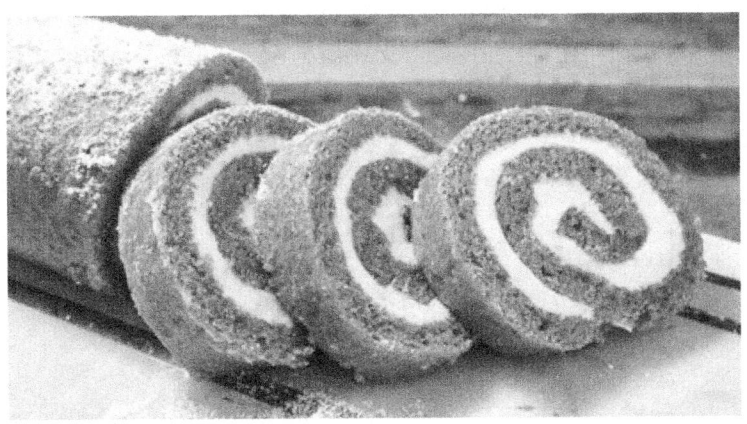

Preparation time: 20 minutes / *Cooking time:* 15 minutes / *Servings:* 10

Ingredients:
- 1 cup sugar
- 3 eggs
- ½ teaspoon crushed cinnamon
- 1 teaspoon baking soda
- ¾ cup flour
- 2/3 cup canned pumpkin
- 1 pinch salt
- 2 tablespoons softened butter
- 8 ounces softened cream cheese
- ¾ teaspoon vanilla extract

Directions:

Prepare a baking tray with greased liner. In a bowl beat eggs, then add ½ cup sugar, baking soda, cinnamon, flour, pumpkin, and salt. Beat and mix all the ingredients thoroughly. In the prepared pan spread the mixture evenly in a layer. Bake it at the 375 degrees preheated oven for 12 minutes. Put the baked cake on the sugar-dusted kitchen towel and roll the cake. Now in a bowl mix the butter, remaining sugar, vanilla extract, and cream cheese. Mix all the ingredients well and spread it in the cake after opening up and again roll it. Cut it into the pieces and serve.

Nutrition: Fats 12.4g, Calories 228, Carbohydrates 27g, Protein 3.9g, Cholesterol 54mg.

Peanut Butter No-Bake Cookies

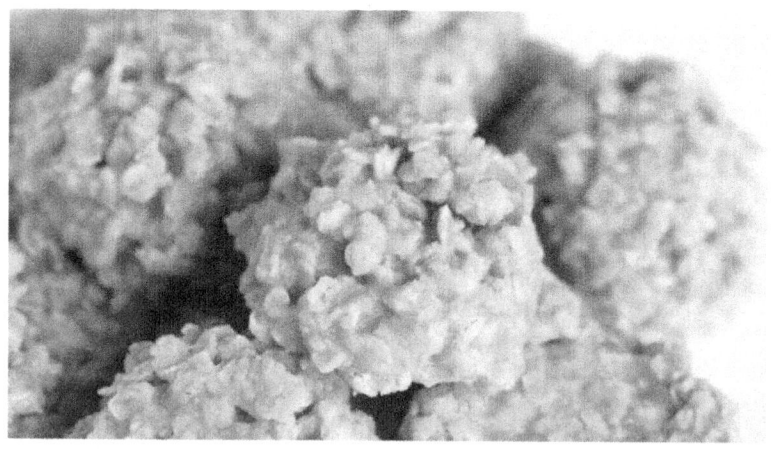

*Preparation time: 05 minutes I **Cooking time**: 05 minutes I **Servings**: 40*

Ingredients:

- ¾ cup soften butter
- 3 cups white sugar
- ½ teaspoon vanilla extract
- ¾ cup milk
- 4 cups quick-cooking oats
- 1 ½ cups soften peanut butter

Directions:

Take a saucepan and add butter, sugar, and milk. Heat it over the medium flame. When it starts boiling cook it for one minute. Now remove it from the stove and add peanut butter, vanilla extract, and oats in it. Mix all the ingredients until they merged and batter starts to cool down. Set the better in the tray in the form of cookies and leave it to cool down.

Nutrition: Fats 7.5g, Calories 152, Carbohydrates 19.4g, Protein 3.2g, Cholesterol 8mg

Apple Pie

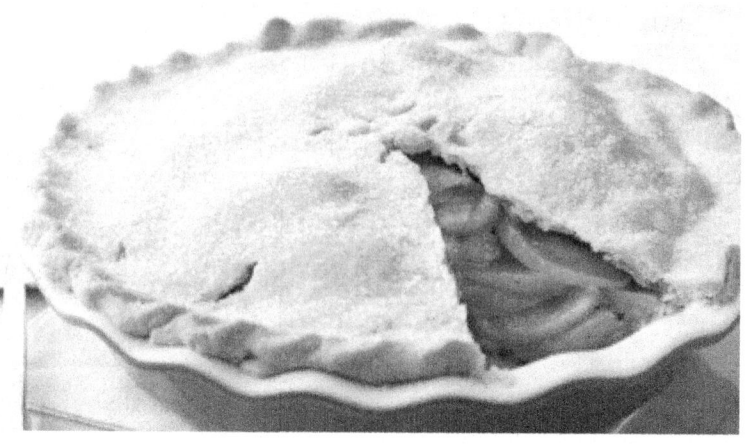

Preparation time: 30 minutes / *Cooking time:* 01 hour / *Servings:* 8

Ingredients:

- 7 cups peeled and sliced apples
- ½ cup granulated sugar
- 3 tablespoons flour
- ½ teaspoon ground cinnamon
- 1 tablespoon lemon juice
- 1/8 teaspoon nutmeg
- 1 double-crust pie pastry
- 1 teaspoon coarse sugar
- 1 beaten egg white

Directions:

In a bowl mix all the ingredients leaving the last three from the list. Take the baking plate and set the double-crust pie pastry in a proper way. Add prepared apple mixture in it. After filling it, cover it from the remaining dough. Seal its edges properly and remove the excess dough. Make small cuts and brush beaten egg white on its top and sprinkle sugar. Bake it in the 425F preheated oven for 15 minutes and after 15 minutes set the temperature at 375F and bake for 40 minutes more.

Nutrition: Fats 12g, Calories 318, Carbohydrates 49g, Protein 3g, Fiber 3g, Sugar 22g

Choco & Fruit Mousse

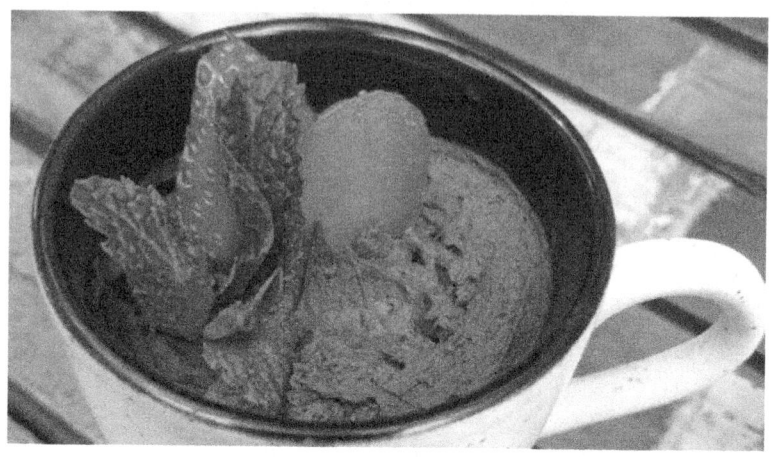

Preparation time: *5 minutes* **/** ***Chilling time:*** *5 minutes* **/** ***Servings:*** *1*

Ingredients:
- 1 peeled banana
- 1 cup low-fat milk
- 1 tablespoon cocoa powder
- 1 tablespoon maple syrup
- 1 tablespoon chia seeds

Directions:
Take a blender and put banana, milk, cocoa powder, chia seeds, and maple syrup and blend it well. Blend it for almost one minute if you have a high power blender. And if you are using low power blender blend it for around 2 minutes. Now pour it in the glass and keep it in the refrigerator for just 5 minutes. If you have to serve it immediately then add ice cubes in it.

Nutrition: Fats 5g, Calories 314, Carbohydrates 68g, Protein 6g, Sugar 32g, Fiber 11g

Chocolate Smoothie

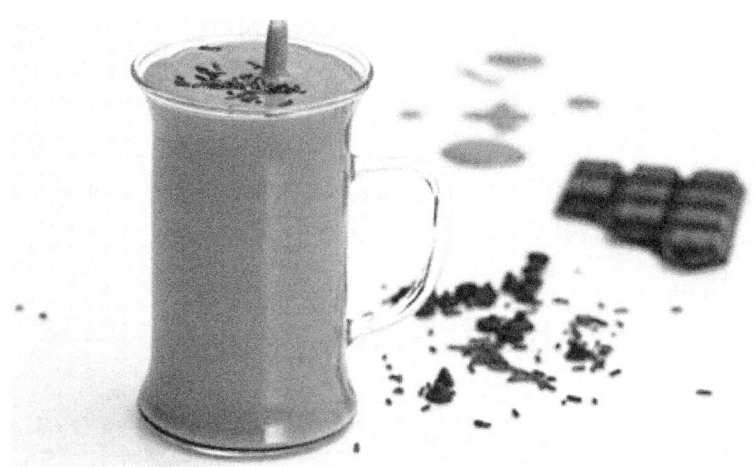

Preparation time: 15 minutes / *Chilling time:* 60 minutes / *Servings:* 6

Ingredients:
- 1 tablespoon sugar
- 2 cups cream
- 5 egg yolks
- 1 tablespoon vanilla extract
- 5 egg whites
- 4 oz. chocolate chunks
- 1 tablespoon instant coffee
- 1 cup fruit sliced fruit of your choice

Directions:
Add cream in a bowl and whip it perfectly. Now add sugar and vanilla extract and blend it well. Melt the

chocolate in a boiler. Take a bowl and add egg yolks in it one by one. Mix it well and leave it for 5 minutes. Take another bowl and stir egg whites and add them in the chocolate mixture. Now take a cup and add fruits in its base (fruits can be kiwis, banana, litchis, strawberry, litchis, and so on). Add chocolate mousse and cream mixture in the cup in the form of layers. Refrigerate it for at least 60 minutes and then serve it.

Nutrition: Fats 38g, Calories 481, Carbohydrates 28g, Protein 8g

Grilled Cheese Bites

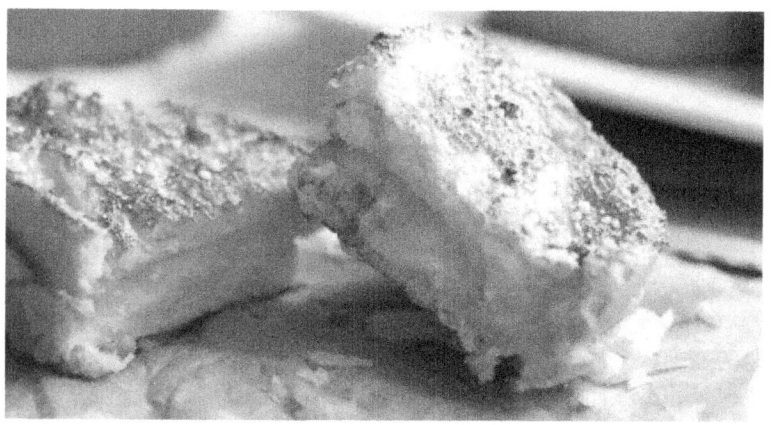

Preparation time: 10 minutes / *Cooking time:* 10 minutes / *Servings:* 6

Ingredients:
- 1 cup grated cheese
- 1 ounce prepared pizza dough
- 1½ tablespoons garlic powder
- 1 tablespoon olive oil

Directions:
Preheat the oven at the 400 degrees F temperature. Roll the pizza dough till the ¼ inch thickness. Make the 24 circles with the help of a jar. Put the small amount of grated cheese on the 12 dough circles and sprinkle garlic powder on it. Now place the plain dough rounds on the rounds with cheese and close it from all sides by pressing it gently. With a brush drizzle, olive oil on each prepared dough bites and place it in the baking tray. Bake it in the preheated oven for around 10 minutes.

Nutrition: Fats 35g, Calories 457, Carbohydrates 31g, Protein 6g

Chopped Chickpea Salad

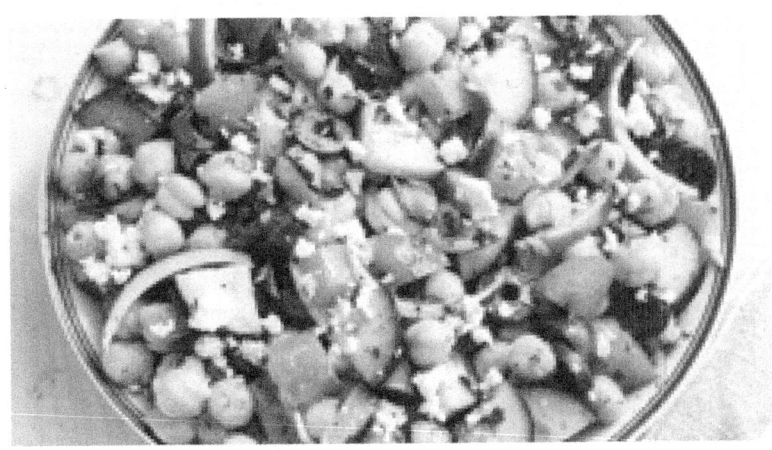

Preparation time: 10 minutes / *Chilling time:* 60 minutes / *Servings:* 4

Ingredients:

- 1 cup rinsed and drained chickpeas
- 3 chopped bell peppers
- 1 cup diced tomatoes
- 1 sliced cut cucumber
- ¼ cup cubed cut onion
- 1 cup shredded cheese
- 1/3 cup sliced olives
- 1 crushed garlic cloves
- ½ teaspoon crushed salt and pepper
- 1 teaspoon dried oregano
- 2 tablespoons lemon juice

- 2 tablespoons olive oils

Directions:

Take a bowl and add olive oil, garlic, oregano, salt, pepper and lemon juice in it, mix it well and set aside. Take another bowl, add all the remaining ingredients in it, and combine them well. In the second bowl add the dressing mixture and whisk it well. Place it in the refrigerator for around one hour. After an hour it is ready to serve.

Nutrition: Fats 12.3g, Calories 279, Carbohydrates 33.5g, Protein 12.5g, Sugar 12.4g

Frozen Berry Yogurt

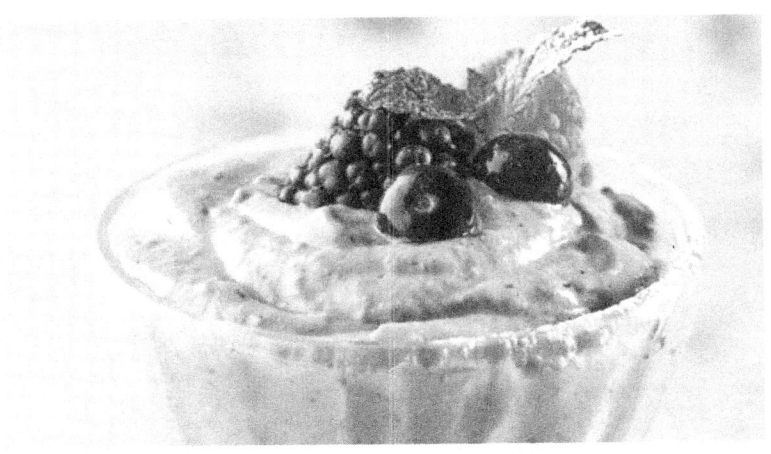

Preparation time: *5 minutes* I **Chilling time**: *3 hours* I **Servings**: *4*

Ingredients:
- ½ cup plain yogurt
- 2 cups frozen berries
- 1 teaspoon vanilla essence (optional)
- 2 tablespoons honey

Directions:
Take a food processor and add all the ingredients. Blend it for 2 minutes or until the ingredients transform in a creamy mixture. Pour it in the ice cream container and put it in the refrigerator for at least 3 hours. Now put it in the serving dish with the help of scoop.

Nutrition: Fats 1.2g, Calories 93, Carbohydrates 20.8g, Protein 1.6g, Sugar 17.4g, Cholesterol 4mg

Choco Bombs

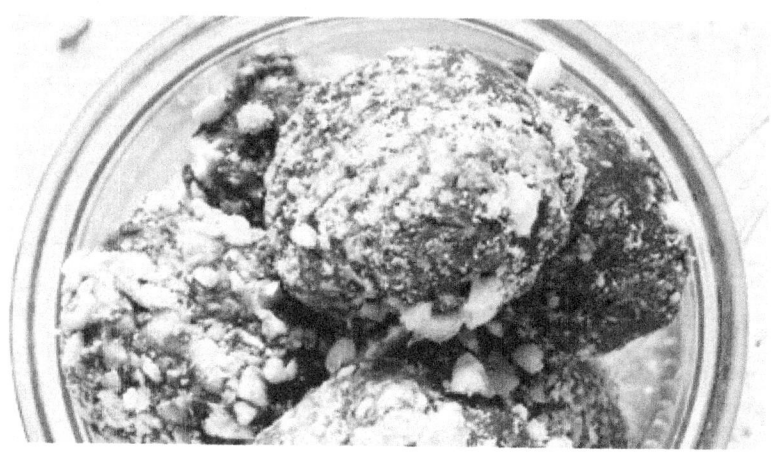

Preparation time: *20 minutes* **/** **Chilling time**: *1 hour* **/** **Servings**: *24*

Ingredients:
- ½ cup white sugar
- 2 tablespoons cocoa powder
- ½ cup margarine
- 2 tablespoons cold coffee
- ½ cup butter
- 1 teaspoon vanilla extract
- 1 ½ cups rolled oats
- ½ cup brown sugar

Directions:

Take a bowl and whisk the margarine and sugar. Add remaining ingredients except the brown sugar, in it and mix it well until all the ingredients merged well. Take the prepared mixture and make small balls. Sprinkle the brown sugar on these balls and put it in the refrigerator for an hour.

Nutrition: Fats 4.1g, Calories 86, Carbohydrates 12.1g, Protein 0.8g.

Chocolate Chip Muffins

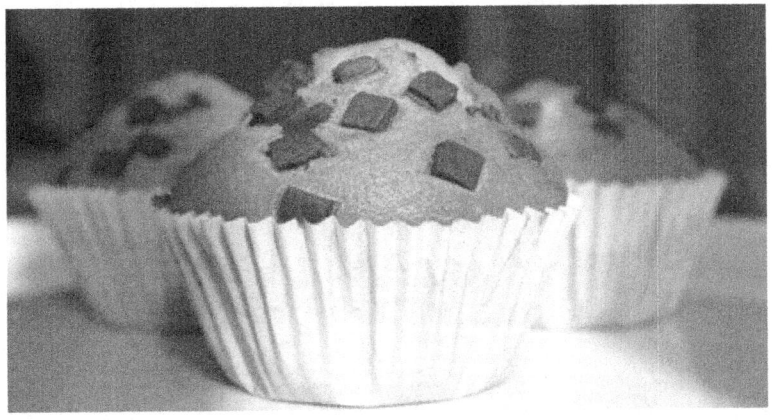

Preparation time: 15 minutes *I Cooking time*: 30 minutes I *Servings*: 12

Ingredients:
- ½ cup melted butter
- 2 eggs
- 2 teaspoons baking powder
- 1 cup crushed sugar
- ½ teaspoon salt
- 2 teaspoons baking soda
- ½ cup milk

- 1 cup chocolate chips
- 2 cups flour
- 1 teaspoon vanilla extract

Directions:
Prepare muffin tins with greased liner. Take a bowl and add butter and sugar in it and blend it well. Add the remaining items in the bowl one by one and stir them well. Now pour the prepared batter equally in the muffin cups. Put it in the preheated oven at the 425 degrees F. Bake the muffins for around 25 to 30 minutes or until a toothpick comes out clean when inserted in the middle of a muffin. Transfer them on the serving plate and serve them.

Nutrition: Fats 8g, Calories 313, Carbohydrates 41g, Protein 4g, Fiber 1g, Cholesterol 49mg

Cinnamon cupcake

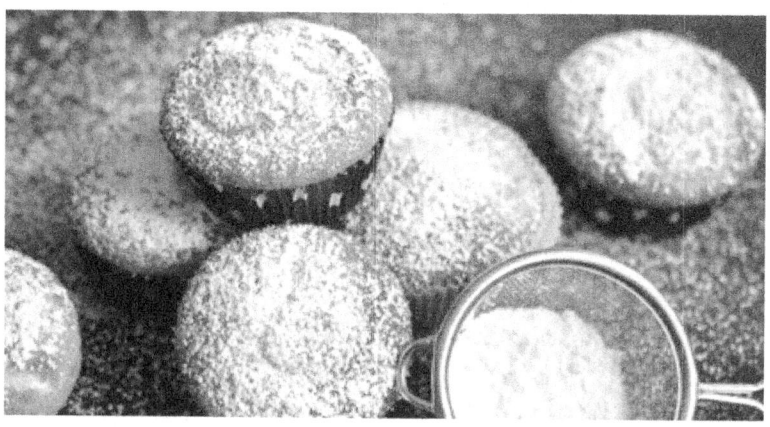

Preparation time: 15 minutes I *Cooking time:* 30 minutes I *Servings:* 6

Ingredients:

- ½ cup melted butter
- 2 eggs
- ½ cup flour
- 1 cup crushed sugar
- 1 tablespoon cinnamon powder
- 1 teaspoon vanilla extract
- 1 pinch cocoa powder
- 2 teaspoon icing sugar

Directions:

Prepare muffin tins with greased liner. Preheat the oven at the 350F temperature. Add butter and sugar in a bowl and mix it well. Now add remaining ingredients in it and mix them well until all the ingredients merged well. Put the batter in the prepared muffin try equally and bake it for 20 minutes. Before serving sprinkle icing sugar on it.

Nutrition: Fats 19.8g, Calories 436, Carbohydrates 63.9g, Protein 3g, Fiber 1.3, Sugar 49.8g, Cholesterol 34mg.

Mixed Fruit Trifle

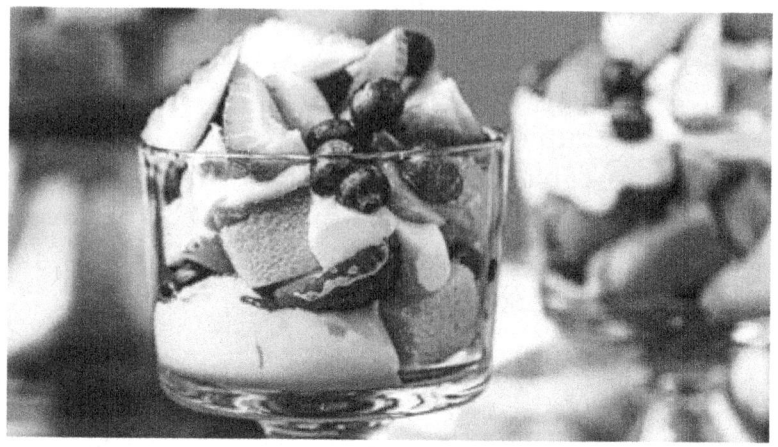

Preparation time: 15 minutes / *Chilling time:* 30 minutes / *Servings:* 4

Ingredients:
- 1 marble cake
- 2 cups milk
- 1 cup banana pudding
- ½ teaspoon maple syrup
- 2 cups whipped cream
- 1 bowl frozen mixed fruits

Directions:

Take a bowl and beat the cream and sugar. Cut the cake in a small diced form. Take a serving bowl and place the cake pieces in its bottom. Add pudding, prepared cream, and fruits in the form of layers. Put it in the refrigerator for 30 minutes for chilling.

Nutrition: Fats 33g, Calories 258, Carbohydrates 55g, Protein 9g, Sugar 27g, Cholesterol 60mg.

Carrot Cake Bliss Balls

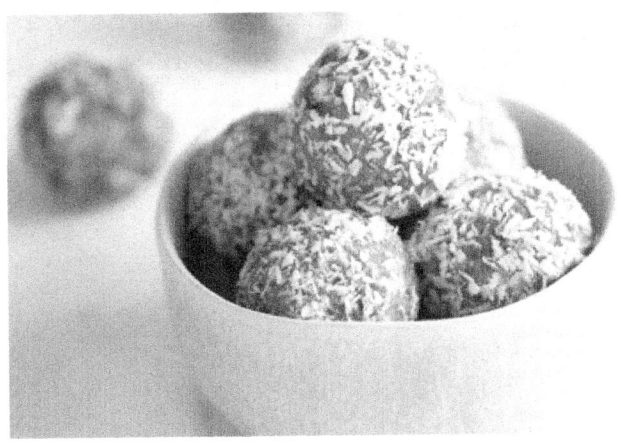

Preparation time*:* *10 minutes I **Chilling time***:
*30 minutes I **Servings***: 6*

Ingredients:
- 1 cup toasted rolled oats
- ½ cup toasted sunflower seeds
- 6 pitted dates
- ½ cup grated carrots
- 1½ tablespoons cinnamon powder
- 2 teaspoon icing sugar
- 1 pinch cocoa powder
- ½ cup shriveled coconut for coating

Directions:
Add all the ingredients in the blender and blend it for around 3 minutes or until all the ingredients are finely chopped and merged well. Take a small

amount of batter in your hand and make a ball. Coat it with desiccated coconut. Store the balls in the refrigerator for chilling for around 30 minutes.

Nutrition: Fats 2.6g, Calories 87, Carbohydrates 15g, Protein 1.8g, Fiber 2.2, Sugar 8.4g.

Chapter 12
21day Meal Plan

Weight gain and obesity are the growing problems that people are facing nowadays. The main reason behind the issue is inactivity and busy schedule, due to which it is hard to streamline the proper food intake. Moreover, because of undue pressure the intake of junk and unhealthy food are getting higher and that turns everyone's life into an unhealthy one. As the weight gain brings multiple of other health complications together like blood pressure, obesity, blood sugar, anxiety, inflammation and many other issues, to deal with these problems many people adopt different ways of dieting, meal plans, fasting tips and workouts. Some are effective, but everything is not for everyone.

Almost everyone has a different body structure and hormones balance, due to every dieting method, it may not give the same results to everyone. Besides all, intermittent fasting is one of the best and popular way to overcome the excessive weight with the healthy way of fasting and eating. Indeed, in this way of losing weight, a person usually breaks out the day into fasting and eating window that provide opportunity to fast between the meals and boost the overall metabolic function.

The body needs energy to perform the functions properly and without the supply of energy in shape of food intake, body switch towards the stored body fats. It starts cutting down the fats into energy and body utilizing that energy to perform the different tasks, when a person is on fasting condition. Some consultant refers that fasting with the workout gives more effective results in less time, and if a person adds the weight training with the fasting, it will definitely boost the metabolism and protect the muscle mass to reduce. Intermittent fasting is the way that almost suits to everyone.

What is mean by meal plan?

Meal plans are most effective and beneficial way to limit the quality food intake with the fasting and eating windows. It is highly recommended that the person should follow the proper meal plans that suits the body requirement.

What about 21-day meal plan?

Eating without thinking may give adverse effect to the health in shape of weight gain. 21-day meat plan is an advanced meal plan that helps to restrict the food options into a specific one. A person who is following the plan has to eat only the listed product that do not need to count the calories before eating, and sometimes for someone even does not need to have a high intensity workout session. In the list of meal plan certain products that are added includes eggs, lean meat, veggies, lemon, lime, limited spices and many other items. Finally, a person has to switch the items each day.

If a person follows the 21-day meal plan with the intermittent fasting method the results will be shown quickly, as it does not only boosts the metabolism but it also helps to keep the stamina and energy level up to the mark.

Things to list down in 21-day meal plan

In 21-day meal plan person has to include only the restricted items that are defined with the low carbs and calorie food items, but they are able to provide a high amount of energy so the body can survive and act confidently. Here is some food that can be included in 21-day meal plan:

- Low carbs or whole food items
- Low fat dairy products
- Lean meat, fish or eggs
- Non-starchy vegetables
- Brown rice or quinoa
- Legume based pasta
- Almond, walnuts and other nuts those are high in fiber
- Unsweetened or unsalted rice cake
- Almond or peanut butter
- Cottage cheese
- Greek yogurt

While making the 21-day meal plan the most important thing that has to be considered is use the minimum amount of salt or spices, since high salted or spices in the food act as the water retention in the body and can be a source to store the glucose in the body.

How 21-day meal plan works?

21-day meal plan can be a part of the intermittent fasting and followed in the eating window parallel to the fasting one; it includes the food items that are low in calorie and carbs that make your stomach full for a longer time and helps to avoid the hunger in fasting time. With the appropriate meal and following this plan, it is easy to keep up the body's energy level and the overall mood is improved. A person does not need to count the calories with following the 21-day meal plan because it is already a set form of food items.

By consuming the low-calorie or low carbs food the amount of glucose is not able to store in the body and to boost the metabolism. By increasing the metabolism stored fats and start turning into the energy, the body utilizes that energy into workouts and performs other activities. Eating less calories can keep the fiber and nutrients requirement complete and could switch the habits towards the healthy one. Everyone can have a different meal plan as per the requirement and after consulting the health consultant.

Is the 21-day meal plan being effective or not?

21-day meal plan consist of the list of healthy food items, that are including the whole food, vegetables and non-starchy and salted product. A person can experience an effective weight loss by following the list of some specific food items included in daily meals for almost 21 days consecutively. This plan has a significant impact on the overall health. Consultants recommend that with this meal plan a person should have to consume more water and avoid the consumption of sugar. It boosts the metabolism function that starts breaking down the stored body fats into energy.

By following this plan with the intermittent fasting, it doubles the benefits and is an appropriate choice for both the men and women. This is remarkable for losing the weight in short time frame with the exclusive benefits. There is no need to follow any kind of intense workouts or trainings with such eating habits. A person can have a lean muscle mass with strength and stamina.

Benefits of 21-day meal plan

21-day plan getting popular because it has multiple of health benefits. Some of them are as following:

Help to lose weight

The purpose to promote the weight loss by controlling the consumption of sugary and salted products. As per the studies, it is significant that by cutting down the consumption of sugary products and salted one it is easy to reduce the weight, as well as to promote the consumption of good fats, fibers and proteins in overall diet.

Healthy eating habits

By fixing the nutritional requirement and focusing more on the fiber and proteins intake, this method leads to a good and healthy eating habits. People who are supposed to follow the diet plan are consciously avoiding the junk, packed and processed food, as well as following the way to cook the healthy and homemade food that are good for the weight loss.

Give portion control encouragement

Portion control and measuring the portion is an effective way to limit the calorie intake and helps to avoid the overeating, which may lead to weight loss. Usually the cups and spoons are used to have a proper and exact measurement of the portion that a person required to consume in one time as a meal.

Indulge exercise in the plan

In 21-day meal plan it is suggested to add the exercise or activity of almost 30 minutes. This is effective and keeps the muscles active and gives them strength, because losing or maintaining weight have a significant importance of the exercise and physical activity into the life. So, it is recommended to follow the exercise for almost 30 minutes daily or four days in a week with the meal plans.

Chapter 13
Faqs

What is intermittent fasting?

Intermittent fasting is an advanced and effective way to make arrangements of having meals and fasting. People follow a proper meal plan window in which they are concerned to have a proper nutritional food and cut down them into segments between eating and fasting. That is all to get the effective benefits to lose weight and follow the healthy lifestyle. People follow different intermitted fasting methods that depends on the requirement and as per their ease. Due to its remarkable benefits, this way of losing weight is getting popular among people around the world.

Is intermitting fasting effective for weight lose?

Yes, this is true. Intermittent fasting is an effective and result oriented way to lose weight, especially for people who are living with the obesity and getting sick of the extra fats and want to have a flt and healthy lifestyle. In this, a person can just divide the meals into portions and have them with fasting intervals. This process improves the metabolism and utilizes the store energy to fuel up the body in fasting time.

What kind of benefits a person can get it from fasting?

Intermittent fasting is no doubt an effective and popular way to be active, fit and to lose weight. It is more recognizable than any other dieting method. Fasting is just not effective to lose weight but is also good for the health improvement, as it helps to improve the blood circulation, metabolism function and reduces the chances of diabetes in the people having obesity. With the fasting inflammation they can be controlled and reduced the chances of heart issue and high blood pressure. Most importantly, fasting improves the hormonal function and improves insulin level in the body.

Is it safe to do exercise while fasting?

Some people think that exercise with fasting may cause issues and is not appropriate, but in reality, it is really good and effective. Having workout session with fasting not only improves the functions but it also helps to get results in minimum time. So, with exercise a person can build stamina and achieve muscle strength as well.

What is an ideal fasting ratio?

There are multiple methods designed by the health consultant for fasting and a person can choose one that suits best, as well as it can be selected with the expert opinion. Usually, the most common and ideal intermittent fasting method is 16:8 that is followed by people who want to lose weight. It means that a person has an 8-hour-eating window in a day with 16 hours fasting. A person can modify and alter the fasting hours as per the body's demand.

Which time is best for workout?

People set their priorities according to the body requirement and the results they are targeting to achieve.

Usually, the best time or the workout is an hour or two before you have a plan to break your fast; in this time, you can have a full advantage and benefit of exercise. The longer you put the gap and wait between workout and having a meal, the more you will be able to get the benefits.

How to spend day with intermittent fasting?

While following the intermittent fasting it is necessary to follow the proper plan and schedule to spend your whole day. So, adjust the workout timing in between the meal window and, if you follow the morning workout session, then do it before two hours of having a meal to break your fast. If you just skip to have morning training session, then it does not matter because you can adjust it in between your day. However, remember that to get the great results, you should follow the fasting plan at least for a month or long.

Is intermittent fasting being safe?

Intermittent fasting is a safe and result oriented way to lose weight and follow the best outcomes to lose weight. It follows a process in which people just cut down the meal intake that leads calorie deduction without the calorie count. With fasting body functions are improved like metabolism, insulin sensitivity and inflammation that gives multiple health benefits, but those who are facing any serious illness or a chronical disease should follow the fasting method by consulting the health consultant.

Can a person build muscle with fasting?

Usually, with intermittent fasting a person can lose the weight and get lean muscle mass. For the gain it does not have any significant results, but multiple fitness trainers suggest different training or high intensity workouts that help to gain muscle mass as well. High level weight training with the protein intake help to reduce the fats and lean muscle, furthermore, weight lifting protects the muscle lose during fasting.

What are health benefits of intermittent fasting?

Most importantly, intermittent fasting helps to reduce the weight and gets a chance to maintain an ideal one, as it is an effective way to have a healthy body and a sound mind. Parallel to this, there are multiple other health benefit a person can enjoy with this, it includes:

- An effective way to lose weight without losing muscle mass.
- It helps to improve insulin level and reduces the inflammation in blood and body.
- Improves the heart health and reduces the risk of heart attack.
- Improves overall strength and stamina and revitalizes the body functions.

A diabetic can fast or not?

Intermittent fasting helps to improve the insulin sensitivity and maintains the optimal level in the body. According to the health consultants' diabetics can follow the intermittent fasting but it is preferred to consult the doctor before starting, because it directly influences the hormonal level, as well as other functions of the body and may cause the risk of hypoglycemia, this means a condition of low blood sugar level due to limited consumption of the calories and nutrients.

Why intermittent fasting getting popular?

The simple and schedule eating habits are good for the health and they maintain an optimal healthy weight.

However, in today's busy schedule it is hard to follow for almost everyone, but intermitted fasting brings it back into the practice, because it is a different and effective way to control the weight and it leads an active lifestyle. Furthermore, it is getting popular because it brings ease and simplicity in life and now you do not need to count calories or prepare a special meal other than routine.

Is it safe to have supplements or a person can take them with fasting?

Yes, you can consume the supplements while having the intermittent fasting. But the most important thing that you have to consider is not to follow high calorie supplements with the meals. Try to use them with the workout plans. Although, instead of having supplements it is preferable to consume high protein and whole food into the meal window, for the better results.

Who should avoid fasting?

Fasting have a significant effect for almost everyone in form of good weight management and health, but not everyone can follow the fasting in same pattern. People with serious health issue have to consult the expert before starting. So, do not follow the intermittent fasting if you are:

- On a medication
- You have diabetes or an issue of low blood sugar level
- You are under weight
- Have low blood pressure issue
- Suffering from any chronical disease
- A woman who is trying to conceive
- Pregnant and breast-feeding woman
- A person who has any digestive problem

What kind of liquids are allowed in fasting?

While following the fasting you should have to add low calorie drinks into your routine. Thus, consume more water and use electrolytes to improve the metabolic process, as well as coffee or tea without sugar or milk can be consumed. A person has to avoid the sugary drinks and carbonated or energy drinks.

Will the intermittent fasting slow down metabolism?

No, that's not true, in fact, intermittent fasting has a good effect on a person's metabolism function, as it not only boosts the metabolism but it also helps to improve the blood circulation. Moreover, it helps to utilize the stored fats as a source of energy that body utilizes during the fasting period and at the time of exercise. Finally, it effectively reduces the weight and helps obesity.

Will fasting cause the muscle loss?

According to the general studies, it is noticed that the intense fasting and high intensity workout may lead to loss of the muscle mass with the weight. To avoid such situation, it is recommended to follow the high intensity weight trainings. Through weight training muscles got the strength and person can improve the stamina; besides, it also prevents the muscle loss and keeps it strong and lean.

Is intermittent fasting safe for women?

As compared to men, intermittent fasting is not highly recommended for women because it can cause the hormonal changes that leads to certain health complications. According to the studies, it is evident that the fasting effects the menstruation cycle and ovulation process as well. That may cause the problems of infertility and other. So, a woman who is looking to follow intermittent fasting to lose weight, it is recommended to consult the doctor and a health advisor first before starting.

What are the top tips to follow during intermittent fasting?

Intermittent fasting is no doubt an effective and most popular way to diet and lose weight nowadays. There are some tips that a person should follow while following the method of fasting. Here are the tips:

- Consume excessive water throughout a day to keep body hydrated
- Listen to the body first and break your fast, if you feel the body is exhausted and it needs energy
- Do not miss any meal from the schedule
- Consume low calorie drinks to fuel up the body
- Be consistent with the fasting and you should follow for at least a month or two to get the remarkable changes
- Choose the healthy or whole food during the eating period of your schedule
- Have low-calorie and low card diet to make your stomach feel full and avoid the hunger during the fasting time period.
- If you have any eating disorder and other chronical health problem, then stop doing the fasting and consult the health consultant first.

Is this being safe for the children as well?

For children, intermittent fasting is not suitable and not recommended to follow because it leads a low nutrients and mineral supply, which can be dangerous for the kids.

Does a person need to cut more calories with fasting?

No, that's not necessary to cut more calories from the meal window while following the intermittent fasting plans, because during fasting it is necessary to follow a proper count of calorie and, if a person stays on low calorie diet for a long time with fasting, it will turn down the metabolism function.

Conclusion

People are considering the ways to lose weight effectively but they don't want to compromise the health and they want effective results that sustain for a longer time. Intermittent fasting brings a blessing into the person's life who is dealing with the obesity, or other weight related issue and was not able to find out a solution to get rid of it. In market multiple of weight loss supplements, diet plans and methods are available and they guarantee slim and fit physique. However, every method or product is not useful for everyone; but that is not the case of intermittent fasting, because it is not a medication or a supplement, it is simply a method or a lifestyle changes, in which a person adopts too fast for the certain time in a day and eats limited and healthy food to get the full health benefits.

There are different methods of fasting and eating that anyone can choose the one that suits the body or as per the requirements. In this fasting procedure consultant suggested to keep the body hydrated and consume more water and non-alcoholic or low-calorie drinks to support the metabolism. Fasting has multiple other health benefits as well, such as: it helps to reduce the risk of heart disease, diabetics, treat the inflammation, which are good for people having insomnia issue and other remarkable benefits. According to few researches the intermittent fasting is not as supported for women as men, because it can change the hormonal balances that lead health complication and other fertility issues in females. However, for a safe zone woman can do intermittent fasting, but with a proper consultation.

People who want to find out the benefits and looking to start the intermittent fasting can facilitate with this piece of literature that will help to identify the methods to do fasting, as well as a person can better find out the best option by reviewing the all-pros and cons and other factors that can influence the better outcomes and much more. Furthermore, this book provides a comprehensive detail about intermittent fasting and the way through a person can start it well to get the maximum benefits out of it.

Jennifer Cook.

Made in the USA
Middletown, DE
13 May 2020

94422780R00245